# SLEEP: A SHIFT-WORKER'S QUEST

*How a nurse achieved regular quality sleep, and how you can too.*

**Matthias Hepworth**

*This book is dedicated to all the workers of shifts, including; emergency services, factory workers, those who work the land and sea, cabin crew, cruise crew, taxi-drivers, single parents, care-givers and those who are simply struggling to get a good night's sleep.*

*To all of you; may your sleep be nourishing, may you awake refreshed and may you be at peace.*

# TABLE OF CONTENTS

# INTRODUCTION

Many people will claim to have 'tried everything' in an attempt to get a good night's slumber, but to be totally honest they probably haven't, as there are so many different areas of sleep to discover. Whether you want to try and change one thing at a time to find out which one works (like adjusting your diet to eliminate problem foods) or whether you are so desperate that you want to try as many things as possible, then this book is for you.

I have arranged things into categories that follow a logical order, but it's not compulsory to read it as such. Either read through the book in its entirety, or dip in out and jump around to find the bits that could work for you; just be aware that the parts that you overlook could be the ones that, once implemented, may well help you out the most.

People often complain about a lack of sleep but rarely do much to change that, so well done for buying this book with a view to improve both yourself and the lives of those around you. Hopefully this will get you firing on all cylinders soon enough, ideally by tomorrow, but keep at it, your sleep will improve, it really will. You are on the right path, so relax and enjoy the journey.

We all know that a lack of sleep makes our irritable and intolerant moments much more dramatic and severe. Many people don't realise that they actually have a problem at all, and often blame others in the process. Therefore, how well are you sleeping is as relevant as your dietary intake and your elimination via bladder and bowels. Sleep deficiency can also affect your ability to learn, focus and react. These deficits can lead to injuries, decreased productivity, and chronic health problems like heart disease, high blood pressure, diabetes, stroke, depression (and other mental health conditions), obesity, and kidney disease (1). In May 2023 the loss of revenue to the UK economy due to Chronic Insomnia Disorder (CID) now stands at £34 billion each year according to Google. If those figures are just due to those who have been diagnosed, and are not counting the average sleepy citizens that are putting in sub-par effort then the economy loss will be much higher than £34 billion. Wow.

The obsession of eating healthily, often at the detriment of either a balanced diet or just being balanced, is called 'orthorexia.' In 2017, the Journal of Clinical Sleep Medicine coined the phrase 'orthosomnia' (2) as the preoccupation with getting healthy sleep has become a worldwide, cross-cultural obsession. I thought insomnia was a relatively recent thing, a post-millennial wave of technology that has stormed in as the rise of the personal telephone has now become ubiquitous, but thanks to Encyclopaedia Googelia it was Dr. Aristotle back in 350BC who first documented the misery of insomnia.

Sometimes you can't put a structure around why you feel so bad or miserable yet you feel permanently jet-lagged. It is like having an autoimmune disorder or an illness like glandular fever where you are being robbed of your energy and joy. A week or so of great sleep will help enormously whether it's a step towards promotion success, developing entrepreneurial mindsets, or to making your first million. When making changes, the logical way would be to change one at a time to discover what works, but if you're desperate, as I have been, try as many as you can and tweak your routine as you go.

Going to bed early is not actually a waste of time. From a work perspective, it is easy to think that if we stay up later, or continue working later, then we'll get more stuff done, whether that be housework, meal prep, office work, online business, etc. However, the opposite is generally true, as we often get to the point where we are so fatigued that a simple task takes far longer because we are just too tired to accomplish them effectively. This is where lists can be really helpful. There are rare times when I am even too tired to wash the dishes, and every other thing that needed doing would be a struggle if attempted, and I know I'd get snotty when it 'didn't go right' because I'm beyond tired, clumsy as anything and ready to turn the air blue with my frustrations. I stop, get ready for bed ASAP and then write a list of the simple tasks that can be knocked out in about 20 minutes in the morning that would have taken over an hour to do if I had attempted to do them that evening. Equilibrium restored, and I am peacefully drifting off into slumber. But it didn't always start that way, and has taken years of tweaking and evaluating to get my beauty sleep.

Aristotle, Socrates, Plato and many others since have all emphasised the benefit of knowing thyself. Once you know how you tick you can find out how to function better. It is bitterly ironic that those who don't give a stuff about anyone or anything seem to sleep the best. I do care, I care very much about some things and I have certainly struggled to sleep over the years. Caring comes from the heart (as does worrying), so I have had to learn to shelve my mental junk in order to unwind and sleep. It can be done. I just needed a little help accepting the things that I cannot change, more courage to change the things that I can, and the wisdom to know the difference. This remains ongoing.

I could set up my own online sleep clinic, evaluate your problem and then charge you a fortune for advice that I provide in this book, 'tailoring it for you'. However, it would be far more beneficial for you to try these different methods and tips so that you can tailor your sleep habits for yourself.

There are lots of online tests and quizzes to complete in order to discover whether you are a poor sleeper or not. So go ahead, take several quizzes, make a spreadsheet of your findings and wallow in analysis paralysis with your data. I adopt a different approach; since you've bought this book then you probably are a poor sleeper anyway, so work through the book to help you to sleep better. Why complicate it?

N.B. Throughout this book I refer to 'experts' and by that I mean the people who have material on sleep already published. I use the term loosely as just because someone has some material published does not make it credible, nor make them an expert. Myself included, but I have actually tried most of the techniques and tips in this book over the decades, and I jolly loathe anyone who says that, *'you should do this or you should do that'* as if implementing their A, B,C formula will work for everyone.

So highlight the book and write in the margins. Use the extra pages at the back to help. Cherry-pick what you think will work, and if they don't, then try some of the other tips. Don't merely think that you might sleep better, but *know* that you will. Believe that it will come to pass from tonight. Declare it out. Fake it until you make it.

# CHAPTER 1
# BEDROOM

At its most basic, we need somewhere to sleep, something to sleep on, and something to cover us. True that there are those who sleep on the floor (which I address later), and there are those who prefer no covers at all, but for the rest of us, we all need some gear. For the true minimalist, you only need the floor, a blanket and a suitcase for your clothes. Other true warriors may opt for a hammock, which is a great minimalist option, but for everyone else, a bed of some form is required.

# BEDS

I understand that many people know everything there is to know about beds, but there will be students and other younger people who don't, so I've included most of the different bed types, along with a brief explanation of the more popular styles.

The simplest way to choose a bed is to look at hotel beds and go for a style that you like. Or you could get ideas from your favourite films. Details like mattresses, bedding etc., will be personal to you, but the overall bed type is easier to find if you know roughly what style you are looking for.

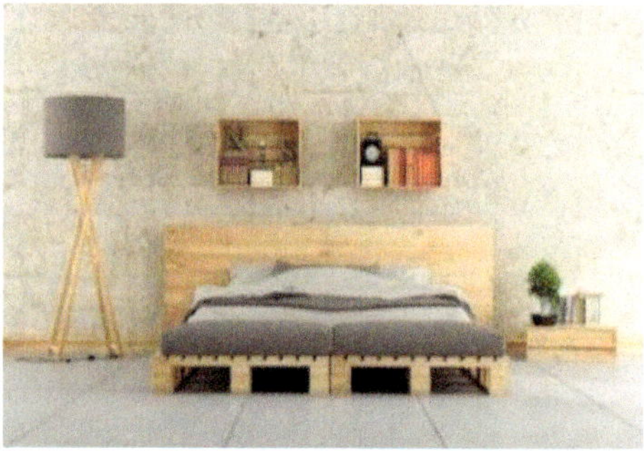

Perhaps one of the easiest minimal bed ideas is simply plonking a mattress on the floor, job done. A slightly more sophisticated approach is to create a platform bed, Japanese style, that is low to the floor. The obvious advantage of these styles is that a bedside cabinet is not required, because with clever design, a pull-out shelf or even a tray will work as a stand for your glass of water, etc.

**Divan beds** are usually smaller than standard bed frames, as the mattress is designed to sit on top of the base rather than in the bed frame. They generally have built in storage drawers that are integrated into the bed base providing under-bed storage, but a word of caution that most are designed to hold clothing or bedding rather than books or other heavy items. Divans can be more durable than the traditional slatted base, as anyone with kids will have found out when they've used it as a trampoline when you've been out of the room. The wooden slats weren't designed for being jumped on!

They sometimes have a box sprung base which is known in the UK as a sprung bed base or sprung base divan. This box spring supports your mattress better than a slatted or hard top base, reducing wear on the spring system contained within the mattress and therefore extending the mattress life.

They often have a headboard that comes with them, but if this is not to your taste then they can be changed easily. If on a budget then they can be made from pallet wood, and laminate flooring can be applied to the headboard, or even to the wall behind to change the image and feel of your room. Very easy to make the room look more modern or rustic/natural using slate grey/black, terracotta or wood effects.

**Platform beds** are a low-profile bed frame with a sturdy base (either solid, metal, or slatted) that holds the mattress up. You don't need a sprung base with a platform bed, so be sure to get the correct mattress for your needs. Platform beds may be too firm for sleepers who prefer a softer, more contouring sleeping surface. There is also a disadvantage that solid platform beds don't allow much air circulation beneath the mattress, so they may create a sleep environment that may be uncomfortably hot for some sleepers. There is also a risk of the underside of the mattress going mouldy if there are no vents or holes in the base.

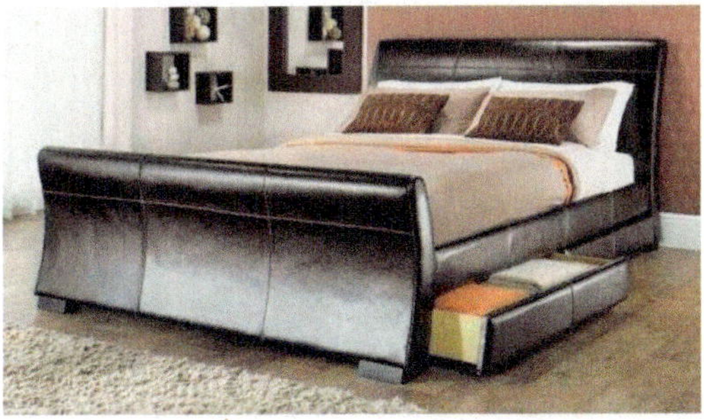

Standard beds generally have a headboard and footboard, and some have storage incorporated underneath.

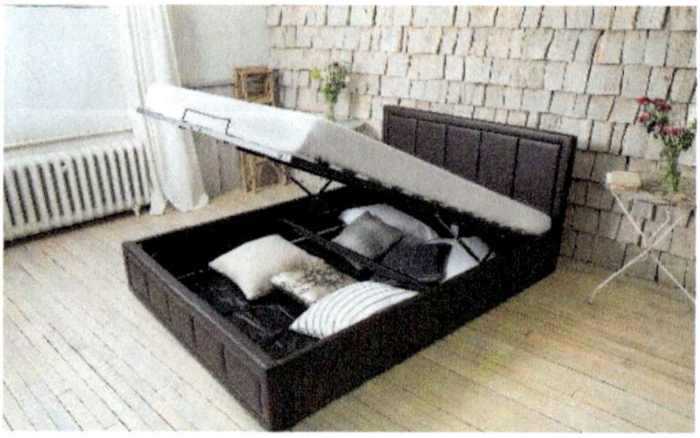

**Ottoman beds** are fantastic for storage, but not so ideal for everyday items. Perfect for out-of-season clothes, bedding, footwear and other miscellaneous items. They usually have gas-lifting hydraulics (as on the rear hatch of a car), but can still be quite heavy to lift. That said, they are not generally opened daily, but the weight is worth noting.

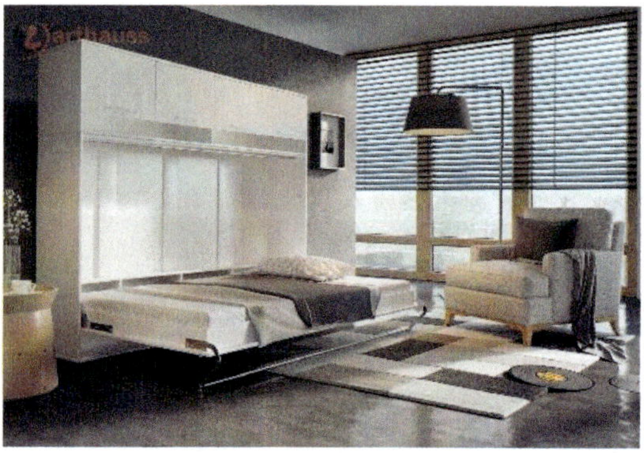

**Murphy beds** are great for studio flats, small apartments and teenage bedrooms. For those that have a home gym, especially if suspension trainers are used from the ceiling, then a murphy bed is handy as it enables a clear floor space to work out. Also ideal for those who do Pilates, stretching or callisthenics, as it provides good floor space to exercise. It must be noted that the duvet and pillows don't always fit away as tidily as the showrooms would have you to believe.

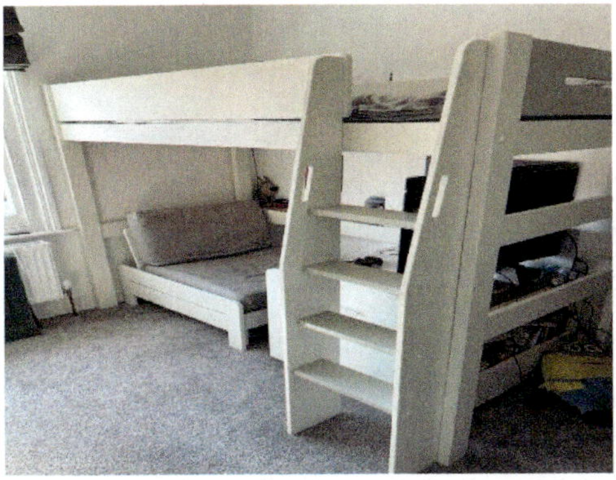

**Loft beds** provide a great space saving solution, and home offices or complete wardrobe storage can be utilised underneath. If storage is your thing, then look up IKEA bed hacks as there are several plans and YouTube tutorials showing some very clever designs using chest of drawers and/or base units as a bed base.

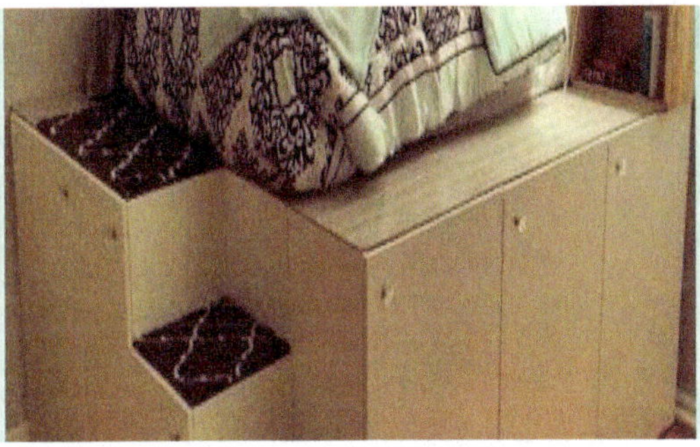

One of the great uses of this idea is that you can put your suitcases, out of season clothes, rucksacks, sporting goods, etc., out of the way until required. They are a good way of utilising otherwise unused bedroom space, and if made correctly, can easily be transported to a new home. If plywood is used as a base, do not forget to add holes to the bed base to allow moisture out and air in, otherwise the mattress may well go mouldy. Been there, it does. A simple 25-30mm spade drill bit should do the trick, and be generous with the holes - but don't get too carried away, just make sure that there is some bed base left.

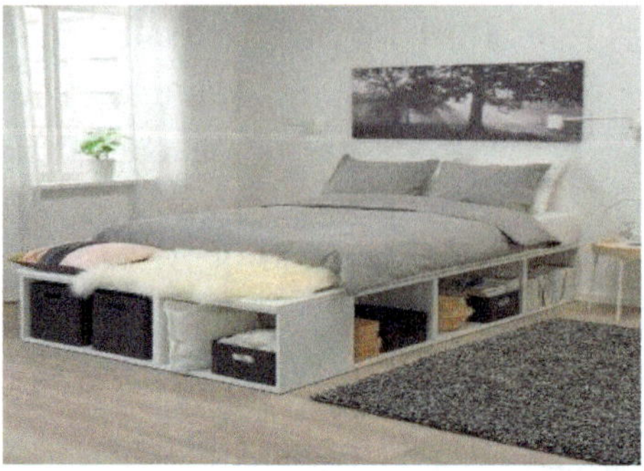

The taller loft beds may not be the best option for those who have the need to wash their hands several times in the night. Caution must also be considered with those who are overly familiar with wine. This design demonstrates a suitable compromise, and by removing the back of the bottom units and using decorative boxes and baskets will provide access to the very centre of the bed which provides excellent storage space.

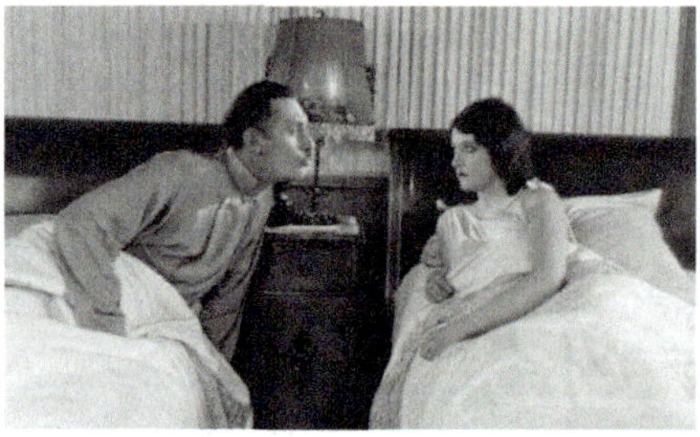

**Twin beds:** If one or both are a lighter sleeper, then two single beds may well be a better option, but it just seems so strange. This concept of a 'sleep divorce' whether it be in separate beds, or even separate rooms can look like a deal breaker but can be a marriage saver. Like everything in a relationship, communication is key.

If one of you goes to bed first, in the spare room, without discussion then it's bound to raise questions. Talk it through, maybe separate beds/rooms could be a temporary fix, as we all go through different seasons in life. Pregnancy and new-borns can seriously disrupt sleep, and preparing for an important interview or starting a new career can require one's sleep to be on point, so there's no shame in a slice of solo sleeping for a period of time. Apparently, according to research, there can be a loss of intimacy from sleeping apart, but by being affectionate throughout the day, through lingering looks over breakfast, to impromptu texts, and then embraces whilst cooking can all, apparently, help to keep some level of intimacy going within a relationship. For some, the notion of a separate bed or room would be a great relief, even if they had to remain in the same house, so just keep telling your partner that it's all for a better night's sleep.

Just bear in mind how necessary sleep is, and if the other person is not getting enough sleep, then they are less likely to have the energy for other things. This can affect the relationship in a whole manner of ways. Single beds can actually be a marriage saver, so don't immediately rule them out. See the section coming up on duvets for an interesting compromise.

However, for the more adventurous there are a many other options. Taking a deep jump down the rabbit-hole of beds there are a few more bed styles that are worthy of a mention:

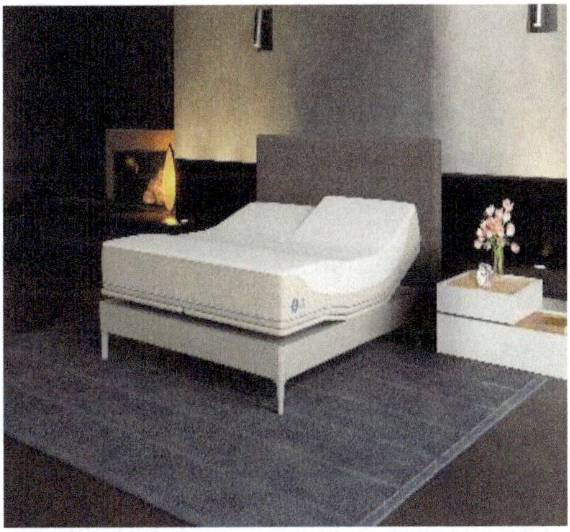

**Sleep Number 360** is sheer technology decadence, that boasts, "when you go to sleep, the bed goes to work". Self-adjusting comfort throughout the night - as you sleep, the bed responds to your movements, adjusts the firmness, allows for side sleeping and alleviates pressure points.

Alleviate snoring - with Partner Snore™ means that you can gently raise your partner's side of the bed, which may alleviate mild snoring. It warms the foot of the bed, creating a cosy feeling so that users can fall asleep faster. It tracks factors that affect your sleep quality, such as your average heart rate, movement, sleep/wake cycles and others, such as regulating your temperature throughout the night. Over time, tracking these factors can help you improve your quality of sleep. This knowledge can be used to help you sleep better.

However, is all this technology really necessary? Each electronic feature has the potential to fail, and not all the Sleep Number 360 beds have the temperature balancing feature. A king size in 2023 was about $12,500 - and they are currently only available in the USA.

**Other bed types:**

- **Day-beds and futons** for guests, children or compact living. The thing that irritates me when these are being advertised is that there is very little mention of where the bedding goes when not in use. You never see the pillows, duvets and PJs stacked in a corner during a magazine shoot. Ever.
- **Scandinavian beds** appear clean and functional, hence the popularity with Ikea.
- **Bookcase bed**; where the headboard forms a bookcase. Beware that dust and clutter may become a problem though.
- **Four-poster beds**, low-poster, half-poster and canopy beds (think lace and voile around the canopies). A healthy dose of Cottagecore would be required within the room.
- **Round beds** - yes, they do exist and are, well, round. Enjoy trying to find bedding for them…
- **Hanging beds** are suspended from the ceiling with ropes, and swing like a hanging garden seat. Perfect for Tarzan and the more agile of sleepers. I simply couldn't imagine getting in and out of bed at 2am from a hanging bed to wash my hands.
- **Rocking beds** are usually flat with a mechanical device that gently rocks the bed to allow you to fall asleep as in your mother's arms - apparently! There are some with a unique

design of being shaped like a large oval, with the mattress in the middle and I assume that they would need some form of manual rocking, by you, whilst you're trying to get to sleep. The thought of having to manually put effort into rocking myself to sleep would probably keep me awake anyway, but for sheer uniqueness they're worth a look.

- **Wave beds** have also got some more unusual shapes. Great for surfers.
- **Rustic, Country and Traditional** beds are all as their names suggest. More Cottagecore required.
- **Sleigh beds**; you don't have to be a fan of Elf to enjoy this style. Wooden or upholstered, they're quite pricey but can really make a room look complete without looking too cluttered.
- **Cottage beds** - think country cottage with lots of Laura Ashley prints. Lovely, dated or chintzy is in the eye of the beholder. Expect to have LOTS of cushions and throws and other paraphernalia with this type of bed! Cottage-core heaven now!
- **French beds** are seen as opulent and usually have curved head and foot boards that often have tufted upholstery with deep buttons. Like the cottage bed, French beds are often 'busy' with accessories, so not ideal if you swing towards minimalism.
- **Rattan, wicker, jute or woven beds** appear very natural and adding macrame ropework around headboards etc. can be quite majestic, so have a look if you're intrigued by the natural look. If you're a bit artsy then you could do some ropework yourself. If you're a bit crafty then you'll trick friends into doing it for you.

- **Standard beds** usually have a headboard and footboard. They may be made of wood, brass, wrought iron (strong, but cold to touch) and upholstered.
- **Adjustable beds** raise the head or feet or both at once, much like a modern hospital bed. Very handy for those who need their head elevated due to breathing problems, acid-reflux etc., or for those who spend long periods in bed. Ditto for those with lower limb problems where elevation is required.
- **Water beds** can help to reduce stiffness which may make you feel more relaxed at the start of your day. Thanks to the even support and pressure distribution there is a greater blood circulation and users are less likely to develop bed sores. When researching waterbeds, to my joy there was a waterbed showroom less than a mile from where I live, so I went to High & Dry Waterbeds in Portsmouth UK to try one out. I'm a slim chap, with very bony shoulder-blades, ischial tuberosities (bony bum when I sit down) and prominent shin and ankle bones, and I can honestly say that lying on the water bed in the showroom was fantastic, like lying on a cushion.

  The staff were very helpful considering that I wasn't there to buy one, and they said that the interesting thing is that they often get several orders to a similar postcode, as someone buys one, boasts about it, and then friends and neighbours try it and decide to get one for themselves. They cost less than £25 per year to heat, and don't get too hot as the temperature can be adjusted; also the mattresses can last up to 20 years as they don't get the usual wear and tear. Easy to clean, therefore very hygienic. Furthermore, they work out less expensive than buying two standard mattresses over a 20-year period. If you can try one at a hotel or showroom then go for it. I currently live alone, but when I don't, we will go and try one together to see how she feels about the idea, as they don't work for everyone. However, many people who try one go on to buy one, and then ask why they are not more popular. I've just got the lava lamp for now.

## Children's Beds

These are really just limited by your imagination. Children can be easy to please, are often whimsical and are generally shorter and more agile than adults, so there are so many options available.

- **Bunks:** classic, triple and built in bunks. Add a slide for fun!
- **Trundle:** where the bed pulls out from underneath.
- **Loft:** with homework office or play area underneath.
- **Treehouse or cabin:** similar to bunks, with the bed at the top or bottom; use your imagination.
- **Novelty:** shaped like a car, rocket, Batmobile, giant sweetie etc. This style is only limited by your budget or imagination. There are a lot of designs that can be made with pallet wood as well (farm, pirate, army, cabin in the woods etc.).

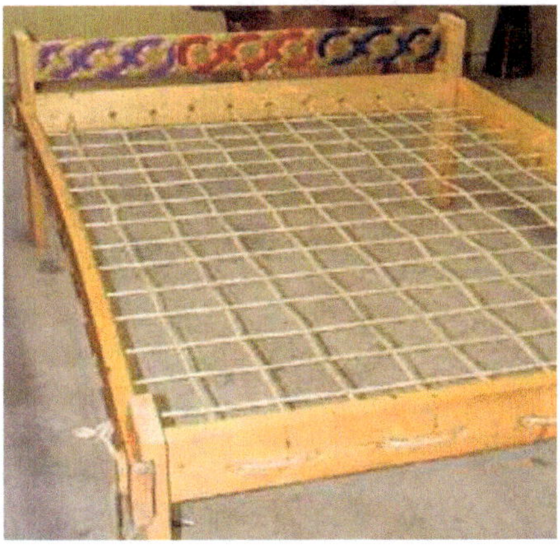

Finally, you can buy medieval types of bed with a wooden base and ropes which need to be kept taut, which is where we get the phrase 'sleep tight'.
But, from corsets to cod-pieces, to avoid a ropey night's sleep, I'd personally leave this slice of medieval history behind.

## HEADBOARDS

These don't require much of a mention, as generally they don't help you get to sleep, but whilst you're thinking of what bed type may work for you it is worth thinking about your headboard too. The entire look of your bedroom can be changed by simply changing your headboard style.

**Feature Walls:** I've seen beds that have simply been pushed up to a wall, job done. Tell yourself 'It's temporary' to feel better about it. It often looks better if said wall is painted a different shade to make a feature wall, but it's not compulsory. Laminate flooring can be attached to the wall to form a feature headboard, or simply attached to an old headboard with some additional timber to enable a removable one.

**Au Naturel:** Driftwood can also be used very creatively to form a headboard. Alternatively, weave branches of willow to form a pattern and shape that you like. Alternatively go all out to create a Lord Of The Rings elven-style bed. If you like it then why not?

**Up-cycle:** Most headboards can be upcycled to some degree, by painting or adding or removing fabric/accessories to create a new image. They can have a simple box framework that can have laminate flooring attached to create whatever effect you desire. Do your research, get creative and enjoy the process.

## MATTRESSES

When choosing a mattress, phrases like 'ultimate comfort' and 'providing luxury slumber' spring to mind. But let's face it, adverts that are not enticing are not doing their job. We are all so different and therefore have different requirements. Go to a bed shop, lie down on a few and go from there. Just make sure that you try as many types as possible, i.e., sprung, memory foam, soft, medium, hard and do try a water bed if you can. Generally, firmer mattresses are recommended for those who are overweight or have back problems. Consider asking your physiotherapist or chiropractor for mattress advice as they may know your body better than you do, but remember that their word is just advice, not law.

Also, bring your partner. Unless you know what you *both* like then you both need to try at the same time, particularly if there is a significant size difference between you. A note of caution with memory foam, it can get quite hot, so if overheating is an issue then proceed with caution, although you can add a wool topper to help regulate your temperature better.

Ideally, before buying any new type of mattress to what you've been used to, call several local hotels / B&B's and ask what mattresses they have, and stay overnight in one that has a mattress type that you are considering. You could do the same with friends and family and make a sleepover evening of it. It is highly unlikely that your local bed salesroom will allow you to stay the night in their showroom, so these can be suitable alternatives.

Buying online is cheaper, this is true enough, but if everyone went to a showroom, tried a mattress, and then bought one online then these shops would cease to exist. I'm not against online shopping, but with many high street shops closing this is worth noting.

**Hybrid** mattresses combine the comfort of memory foam and the back support of a pocket sprung mattress, so they offer the best of best of both worlds. This combination of materials reduces the movement felt from one side of the mattress to the other, making them a good choice for couples. They are designed to be highly breathable, helping individuals remain cool throughout the night. The hybrid is best for side sleepers, front sleepers, people who have allergies and people who tend to overheat at night.

**Memory foam** mattresses are designed to contour to a sleeper's body, to relieve pressure on joints and to help to maintain posture by aligning the sleeper's spine. They are recommended for those who need support or suffer from a bad back. They are hypo-allergenic, so good for people who suffer from allergies. They also absorb movement, helping sleepers get better rest, especially if either of you is restless. Memory foam mattresses are good for back & front sleepers and they provide back support. Not everyone finds them supportive for their back, with many people opting for a firm mattress as they don't like the 'sagging' feeling of memory foam. They also get very hot, and many people don't like them for this reason.

**Foam** mattresses include latex foam and cooling gel. These are a budget-friendly option. They feature hypo-allergenic properties, such as blocking pollen and dust mites. They are good for side, back and front sleepers, plus they offer some back support.

**Pocket sprung** mattresses contain individual springs within the mattress that form small pockets which move separately from each other. The number of individual springs can vary from mattress to mattress, with a higher spring count usually being a higher quality mattress. The individual springs help distribute weight evenly, absorbing each person's movements which generally limits one sleeper from disturbing the other. They are designed to adapt and contour to the individuals' bodies, helping support and relieve pressure on joints and backs. 1000 sprung is the basic standard; anything below or above will denote the quality of the mattress, with 2000 being considered a luxury.

**Open coil** mattresses are a basic traditional mattress which features internal springs that are connected by wire and covered with fabric. They are often chosen as orthopaedic mattresses due to generally being extra firm mattresses; they often feature additional elements to improve comfort and durability. They are easily the most affordable option for a new mattress. They are highly supportive and often prioritise firmness. Great for small budgets and lightweight sleepers, so a popular choice for children's beds.

**Wool** mattresses are the traditional choice in the UK and remain very popular. They are breathable and regulate temperature well. They are pretty much chemical-free so no 'off-gassing' like you may get foam mattresses (see the summary in the next chapter for more details). They tend to be combined with pocket springs, and as they are a luxury mattress then most companies will offer a trial period from 30-200 nights, and if you're not happy then you can exchange it for a different type of mattress that the company makes.

| | | |
|---|---|---|
| Single | 6ft 3" x 3ft | 190cm x 90cm |
| Twin | 6ft 3" x 3ft 2" | 190cm x 96.5cm |
| Twin XL | 6ft 8" x 3ft 2" | 203cm x 96.5cm |
| Small double | 6ft 3" x 4ft | 190cm x 120cm |
| Double | 6ft 3" x 4ft 6" | 190cm x 135cm |
| King | 6ft 6" x 5ft | 200cm x 150cm |
| Super King | 6ft 6" x 6ft | 200cm x 180cm |

There are smaller mattresses 6ft x 2ft6" (183cm x 76cm) which are handy for very small rooms, caravans, campervans, boats etc. There are also toddler mattresses at 4ft6" x 2ft3" (140cm x 70cm) available. That said, there are plenty of places online to shop for foam which can be cut to the size that you require.

Regarding toddler mattresses, my children went straight from cot to single bed. They did look kind of funny in a bed that was enormous compared to them but they adapted and all was well. We just kept their cot duvets until they got used to the bed, and then single duvets shortly afterwards.

It's a good idea to change your mattress every 5-10 years. Again, try a shop first, as your preferences may change over time. If your partner sleeps like a stone then you have priority here. Whichever of you is the grumpier of the two without sleep should get the top priority anyway. Buy the best that you can afford, as you spend a third or more of your life on it. Consider a mattress protector. These can be washed to reduce dust mites. Vacuum over the top of the mattress at least every quarter, ideally monthly or more. You may be surprised at what you thought was a clean mattress, how much dust/mites etc. can be seen if you have a powerful vac with a clear cylinder.

## PILLOWS

Experts state that a lack of support for the head and neck during sleep has been found to severely impact spine alignment, and cause muscle stiffness, with problems leading to neck and shoulder pain. However, it is vital to avoid the problem of 'too much' support as you may be killing your body with kindness. For smaller people, particularly children, having two pillows gives too much height so that the head is raised up on the pillow, causing neck strain by default. Realistically the pillow is only supposed to support your shoulder gap between your head and the mattress when you are lying sideways, so it may be time to ditch that second pillow. If you choose wisely then one pillow is usually enough - great news for the minimalist. There are many types of material to choose from, so I have highlighted a few which fall into two categories, synthetic and natural.

**Synthetic** pillows are generally made of polyester and are soft and lightweight. These are cheap to buy and are generally hypoallergenic and hold their shape well. Other synthetic pillows include memory foam pillows and shredded foam pillows, some of which are adjustable, meaning that there is a zip on the end and you can add or remove filling to suit your personal requirements.

**Microbead** pillows as the name suggests, are filled with tiny polystyrene beads, like flight pillows. They are very breathable and hypoallergenic, but good luck trying to clean them up if a pillow bursts!

**Water** pillows are simply filled with water and job done. They may be too firm and non-contouring for some, although I haven't tried one personally.

**Gel** pillows are a cross between foam and water pillows, with a gel strip on top of a memory foam base.

**Air** pillows get the briefest of mentions because it is generally hard to find one large enough for a bed, as they are usually made smaller for camping, and they are what they are.

**Feathers** are the traditional choice for natural pillows, with 'down' feathers being from the chest area of the bird. Down feathers are more favourable as a normal feather pillow is likely to have quills which may poke through the fabric causing discomfort. Down pillows are soft and comfortable and tend to last longer than synthetic ones. Not all feathered pillows are created equally, as the prices will reflect, and some people prone to allergies may not find them suitable.

**Wool** is the other non-vegan filler on this natural list, although the sheep are sheared for their own comfort and wellbeing. It is naturally antibacterial, antimicrobial and regulates temperature well (just ask a sheep for more details). They may flatten quicker than polyester pillows, but can be plumped up again, and can be washed in a regular washing machine using a wool wash detergent. They are generally more expensive, due to processing, but are certainly an all-natural, luxury item. For those wishing to avoid man-made products then they are perfect.

**Latex** is a natural material, but some pillows may have been mixed with polyurethane foam, so watch out for 'blended' on the label. Latex pillows tend to be hotter than others and would obviously not be suited for someone with a latex allergy.

**Cotton** is not common for a pillow filler, but it is a natural material, can be organic and is naturally hypoallergenic and is breathable. The downside is that they can get lumpy over time.

**Kapok** is another natural filler, using seed pod fluff not dissimilar to bulrushes.

**Buckwheat** pillows are filled with buckwheat hulls, which are the hard outer shell that protects the buckwheat seed. The hulls are breathable**,** hypoallergenic and conform to your head and neck to help keep your spine aligned, not dissimilar to microbeads.

*N.B. I have used a buckwheat pillow full-time for the last few years. I was concerned about the swooshing noise as the hulls move in relation to my own movements, but it really doesn't bother me (and I'm picky about noises). In fact, they helped drown out any slight street noises and I told myself that it was 'just the pillow' and tricked my mind into ignoring any slight disturbances.*

The brilliant thing about the buckwheat pillow is that they mould to the shape of your head and therefore stop you tossing and turning quite as much. Even if your head moves just a little, your body will often rotate with it. However, the buckwheat prevents those micro-movements from turning into a complete body change of position and so you get a more restful night's sleep. I can vouch for this one hundred percent.

**To summarise**, synthetic materials such as polyester are comfortable, cheap, and readily available. Other synthetic materials have their merits, as some people swear by the memory foam pillows that provide the orthopaedic benefit for their spine.

However, many have been sprayed with flame retardants such as bromine, chlorine, phosphorus, nitrogen, metals, or boron, which they don't add to the flame-retardant label. There is also a phenomenon known as 'off-gassing' whereby the airborne release of chemicals in vapour form is noted as an odour. Obviously, it happens the most when a product is new. That said, the thought of inhaling the chemicals of a foam pillow does not appeal to me, nor do polystyrene microbeads or plastic covers that hold gels in situ.

Natural pillows, by contrast are made with natural materials which have been around for thousands of years. They tend to be more breathable than synthetics, so are better for temperature regulation. Most natural material pillows will need some form of fluffing up to keep them plump and ready for slumber, but this can form part of your morning routine without much issue.

Do try different pillow types. Buckwheat pillows cost between £20-£30 which was far more than I was used to paying at the local supermarket for a pillow, but I figured that it could be used as a sofa cushion if it didn't work for me, or could be given away to someone else. However, it worked so well that I'm in no hurry to return to standard pillows, and that was over five years ago.

Incidentally, my mother has had several operations to her neck, with metal plates around some of the bones, and like me, she was sceptical at first. Thankfully she decided to give it a go and finds it very comforting as the pillow moulds to the form of the head/neck and gives her the support that she requires.

TOP TIPS: Use two pillow cases on each pillow to keep the pillow fabric clean and stain free. If you machine-wash certain pillow materials (usually polyester) then be prepared for them to go lumpy and be very uncomfortable. However, if you hang them on a washing line to air; twice a year will suffice, but once you enjoy the fresh smell then quarterly or even monthly becomes more favourable. You can even 'trap' them in an open window either by their corner or just resting them there (caution if windy) and they will freshen a bit. Sunshine is naturally anti-bacterial so they will definitely smell fresher. Try it.

Remember that you can always use a pillow that you bought and didn't like as a sofa cushion or keep it in the car for emergencies/children etc., so don't be put off by trying a new style, they can always be given away if not used and you might just strike slumber gold for yourself with that new pillow.

# DUVETS

For clarification purposes, duvets, comforters, quilts, eiderdowns (named after the eider duck) and doonas (G'day mate) will all be collectively called duvets.

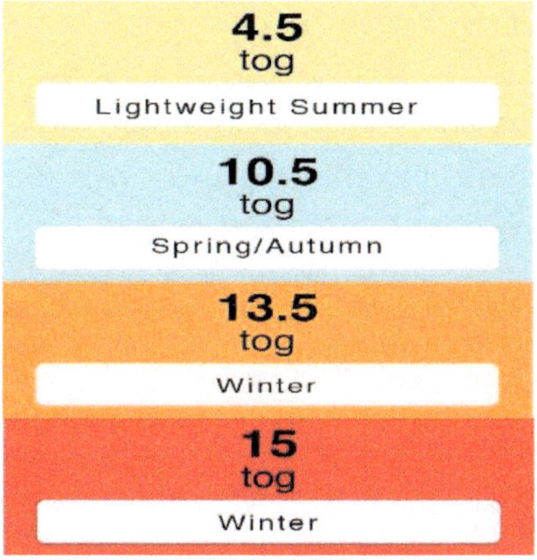
4.5
tog
Lightweight Summer
10.5
tog
Spring/Autumn
13.5
tog
Winter
15
tog
Winter

The tog rating of a duvet is the measure of how the duvet retains heat. Essentially it measures how warm it will keep you throughout the night. The tog ratings range between 1 tog to 15 tog. As per the chart, the higher the tog the better the heat retention (3).

The **fill power** gives the duvet its fluffiness, and the higher the fill power, the better the duvet. It can range from 450 to 900 with good fill power being 600 CUIN and above (cubic inches per ounce). For down duvets, 700 CUIN is the highest fill power for feather duvets.

**Synthetic fibres** are made from a form of plastic, with hollow fibre being the best insulator. They are hypoallergenic and wash well. They are cheap to produce, hence why you see them readily available in supermarkets. Recycled plastic bottles are melted into plastic pellets and spun into polyester fibres. They may be labelled as re:down or r:PET. However, they may release microplastics into the water system when washed. They will also end up in a landfill when disposed of.

**Feather** duvets have a better thermal insulation than synthetic fibres, and so are more expensive. There is a 'Responsible Down Standard' and a NOMITE certification to ensure that you sleep better at night knowing that the feathers are ethically sourced and a by-product of the food industry, and that the duvets are suitable for house dust mite allergy sufferers.

**Wool** filled duvets are breathable, moisture-wicking, hypoallergenic and incredibly temperature-regulating and have the ability to transform your sleep. Sheep are a big fan of wool and they settle down and fall asleep in the process of counting each other.

Natural fillings such as down, feather and wool, are biodegradable, take less energy to produce unlike synthetic fillings, and obviously they don't contain plastic microfibres.

That said, all duvets and pillows that you wish to discard could be donated to an animal shelter to at least get a bit more use out of them.

Downafresh
Hygiene according to DIN EN 12935

NOMITE

OEKO-TEX®
CONFIDENCE IN TEXTILES
STANDARD 100

Downafresh is the European standard EN 12935 for feather and down hygiene and cleanliness.

The NOMITE is the standard for house mite allergy sufferers.

The OEKO-TEX logo verifies that the item is tested against harmful chemicals or toxins.

**Standard UK Duvet Sizes**

| | | |
|---|---|---|
| Single | 4ft 5" x 6ft 7" | 135cm x 200cm |
| Double | 6ft 7" x 6ft 7" | 200cm x 200cm |
| King Size | 7ft 4" x 7ft 3" | 225cm x 220cm |
| Super King Size | 8ft 6" x 7ft 3" | 260cm x 220cm |

**Ring stitching,** also known as "button-tufted," is a construction technique that uses subtle circle-shaped tacking at regular intervals that creates a uniform, decorative pattern. It is favoured for synthetic duvets.

**Quilt stitching** AKA square stitching is favoured for feather duvets.

The stitching is there to prevent the stuffing from moving about or clumping together, resulting in a more even temperature without your duvet looking as if a giant snake has swallowed a pig or that you have a bean bag over your belly with your feet exposed to the elements.

Marriage can be a hot and cold affair, especially in the bedroom, but here I am talking about thermoregulation. If one of you is like an oven, and the other is like an iceberg then you'll have a problem.

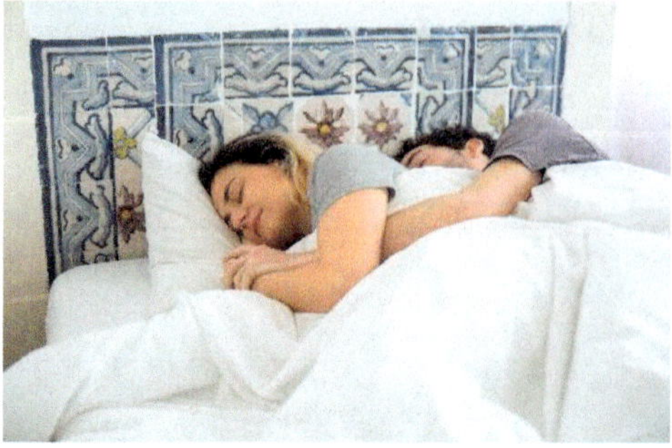

The idealistic solution would be to cuddle up to each other all night, causing a wonderful thermoregulated bliss.

But there is a more realistic way…

## The Scandinavian way

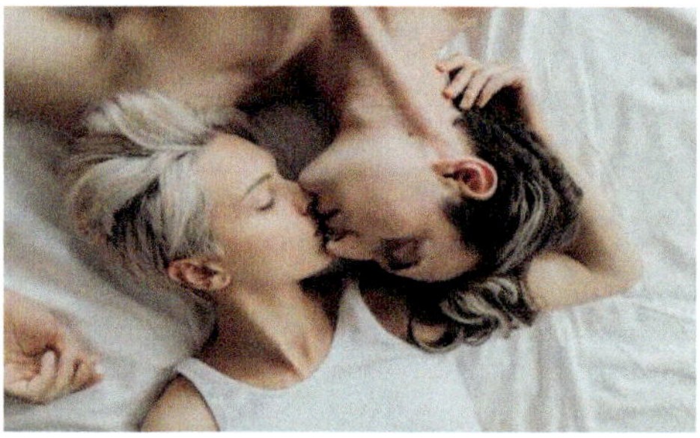

The Scandinavian sleep scenario is one that incorporates two duvets over the same bed.

***Voilà, absolute genius.***

No more tug-of-war to claim the lion's share of the duvet. No more waking up frozen at 2am, or worse still, your partner waking up and claiming that YOU nabbed the duvet overnight resulting in them being grumpy, you ending up with the cold shoulder and both of you being miserable all day.

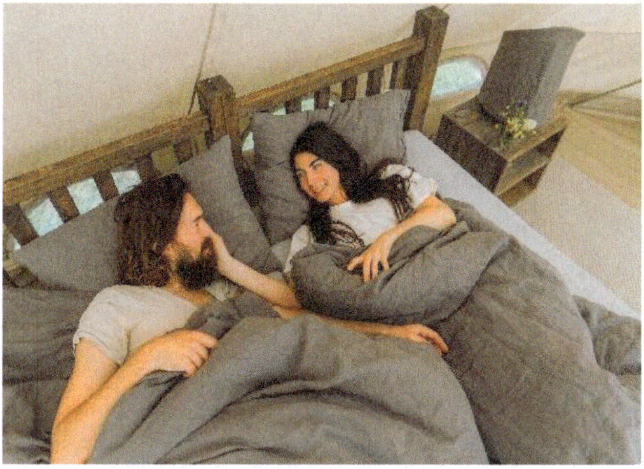

The genius of separate duvets is that you can each choose the weight and type of duvet that works for YOU. I always assumed that couples just shared one duvet, but when I heard of the 'Scandinavian' way of having two duvets on the same bed I was surprised by such a simple solution to an age-old problem.

So, you go to bed either separately or at the same time and then hunker down under your own duvet, the one that YOU chose which is perfect for YOU. Anyone who has had the duvet removed off them by a partner either being over-zealous with their share of it or simply being asleep will know that this is no joke, and for those who struggle to get back to sleep then this is a very real problem - but not any more!

In the morning, simply fold back and re-arrange your duvet at the bottom of your bed when you get up. If you simply buy several white single duvet sets (to avoid the colour clash between Hulk and Barbie) then you can add a touch of colour by adding a throw to cover them both during the day.

## BLANKETS

Blankets are considered 'old school,' and they are, but they are still a suitable alternative to the standard duvet. Blankets have the benefit of layering - just use one blanket in summer but use two or three in winter. A three-layered blanket set-up will usually be warmer than a duvet, although that obviously depends on the duvet tog. The benefit here is that blankets can be added or removed to regulate temperature. The other benefit is that extra blankets add weight, which can help the sleeper to feel more 'grounded'.

Hospitals and old-school care homes have always used blankets, with duvets being the favoured choice in care homes today. Some hospitals are favouring duvets now, but I have a problem with the issue of hygiene between patients. I know that I cleaned the duvets thoroughly after each patient had been discharged, but I certainly cannot say that all other hospital workers did the same.

Mexican blankets (also known as Aztec blankets due to their distinct pattern) are made of wool, and their patterns make them an ideal starting point for choosing colours or accessories within a room. Their general size is about 4ft x 7ft (1.2 x 2.3m), although if you shop around there are many different sizes available.

They wear really well, the one that I bought at a festival in 1996 is still going strong today. Another great thing about them is their weight, as my 4ft x 7ft weighs about 2kg (4lb 6oz) and makes a nice duvet overlay in winter, and the weight is surprisingly reassuring and comforting.

They are hard-wearing and versatile, so can be used at the beach or park, and make a striking throw over a sofa which is also great to snuggle under whilst watching a film in the middle of winter. It's kept me warm Bodhi-style (Point Break) whilst checking the waves, and is a welcome addition on my lap as I write. I am considering cutting a slit in it for my head, to enable me to wear it poncho style, but it will need a serious amount of stitching around the cut to prevent fraying, and I'd jolly well better pick the right place for the opening first, otherwise it will definitely be an 'instant regret' moment. Maybe next year…

Top-Tip. When washing my large Mexican blanket, I simply bunged it in my washing machine. I could have (and probably should have) used wool-wash soap, but I didn't have any, so I used baby shampoo instead; it is soft and mild with no harsh chemicals in it. I used about 50-70mls, but it's not an exact measurement. Try it, it worked well for me, the blanket smells nice and there were no more tears either.

## WEIGHTED BLANKETS

According to a study done back in 2015, the 32 adults that used a weighted blanket, 63% reported lower anxiety and 78% preferred the weighted blanket to calm down. Essentially, weighted blankets have shown positive improvement in sleep and stress levels for people suffering from anxiety (4). But even if you don't have anxiety, some occupational therapists say you'll still feel good under a weighted blanket.

It is common knowledge that anxiety and insomnia are closely related, and research proves this to be true (4). The vicious cycle comes when the overly tired person is anxious to get a good night's sleep, which prevents them from sufficiently relaxing to actually fall asleep, and then the cycle continues. I feel your pain.

Enter the weighted blanket. I first came across these back in 2017 when I was working on a SEND (Special Educational Needs and Disabilities) unit as a teaching assistant whilst taking a year out from nursing. One of the students became unsettled and was having an anxious moment, when a large navy blanket was brought out and he said, 'Yes' and it was then draped over him. I asked what it was all about, seeing the staff member struggle to put it over the lad. The staff explained that it helped with keeping the individual feel grounded, therefore reducing his anxiety.

I wasn't convinced, but he did settle down into story time, so I was intrigued enough to request 'a go' later. Later that day I wrestled this thing over me, my mind racing to see if this was the panacea that society needed. Whilst I was wondering whether the NHS would consider changing benzodiazepines for blankets when I began to notice a change happening inside of me.

As usual, my mind was racing, but I really did feel calmer. The fact that I couldn't move around easily kept me still, which in turn, relaxed me. I am never relaxed when people are standing around watching to see my reaction, but the blanket really did calm me down. Critics compare it to getting a hug, which I cannot, for a hug is underrated as an all-round mood enhancer, but weighted blankets are pretty good at creating a relaxing feeling, and now I know what they mean by feeling 'grounded'.

## BEDDING

Whilst a top sheet is an obvious requirement when sleeping with just blankets, some people favour a top sheet as well as a duvet, but is it necessary? In short, no. However, it does allow for the duvet cover to be changed less frequently if that works for you. The main drawback to the top sheet is that it can get so ruffled up that it ends up out of one side of the bed or by your feet, and is another thing to think about when making the bed. They are best suited for those who don't move about too much, for those who struggle to change duvet covers due to health/mobility issues or for those who like to have regularly washed bedding without the headache of changing the duvet cover so frequently. Cotton is the general go-to for bedding, but don't rule out linen as it is an excellent choice for luxury bedding. It is both durable and hypoallergenic and is ultra-breathable, keeping you cool in summer and warm in winter.

**Cotton** is the most popular material for bed sheets. The best is 100% Egyptian cotton. If a label simply says, '100% cotton' then you can assume that it's not Egyptian cotton, and is made from a rougher, less expensive variety. Luxury hotels tend to use 100% cotton with a thread count of over 300 as they remain affordable, are breathable and can withstand commercial washing. The higher the thread count the softer, smoother and denser the sheet. They are also more durable, and therefore more expensive.

Whilst cotton/polyester is the most common, there are also cotton/rayon, cotton/bamboo, and nylon/polyester. Blended fabrics are generally inexpensive, durable, and wrinkle-resistant, making them a good choice for children's bedding. Terry towelling is made of high-quality terry material of 75% cotton and 25% polyester. They are both cool in summer and warm in winter.

**Satin and silk and velvet**

So, what is the difference between satin and silk? Silk is more expensive, but with good reason. Silk is more luxurious as it is a natural fibre, generally sourced from mulberry silkworms therefore the whole process is more costly. Silk is also more durable and breathable than satin, and is good for both hot and cold temperatures.

Satin is a synthetic fabric, and can be manufactured from a range of fibres, including polyester, rayon, viscose, acetate, cotton and also silk fibre. Different fibres can be woven together and therefore the quality and price of satin is related to the blend. Sleepers sensitive to overheating may get on better with silk, depending on the climate.

Both silk and satin are very good materials for your skin as they allow your skin pores to breathe which may help in the reduction of acne. Contrastingly, if you are prone to dry skin then both silk and satin can also help. In case you've got the song, 'Satin Sheets' in your mind then it was recorded in 1973 by Jeanne Pruett and the song became her biggest hit. Tammy Wynette released her version in 1974, and then Dolly Parton in 1996. That'll save you some doomscrolling on your phone to check!

Velvet sheets are similar to polar fleece but smoother. They are generally made of polyester or another synthetic material, and both are noted for their warmth and comforting feel to them. There is such a thing as pure silk velvet, although it is rare and extremely expensive, so enough said.

**Fitted sheets** are cheap enough, and they stay in place better than a flat sheet, particularly if you fidget a lot at night. They are also quicker to put on and generally remain wrinkle-free. The main reason why hotels use flat sheets for top and bottom is because it's easier to have flat sheets for everything, and they can be fed through a commercial laundry press whereas a fitted sheet cannot, so now you know.

When I'm working on hospital wards, I have a real problem with sheets being tucked in at the bottom of the bed. Agreed, it 'looks neater' but I have had numerous arguments with healthcare staff over the years about making a patient's bed and tucking in the bottom sheet as this causes plantarflexion (excessively forcing the toes downwards), causing ankle strain and can also lead to pressure damage on the toes (due to lack of circulation at the point of contact with the sheet). This is exacerbated by pre-existing conditions (poor circulation, lack of mobility, leg ulcers etc.) which can make the patients lower limbs much worse, all because of a sheet being tucked in. Generally, the healthcare workers state *'I hadn't thought of that'* or *'but we've always done it this way'* or, *'It makes the bed look neat'*. So, if you do use a sheet, or make a bed for someone else, please bear this in mind!

**Washing** Some will advocate washing daily, some weekly, some monthly etc. There is no hard and fast rule for this, just don't leave bedding for too long.

For duvets, pillows, blankets, throws etc. wash when they get gross, icky, yucky, grubby, manky etc. Air them as often as possible, unless you like regimented cleaning routines; if so, type up an Excel spreadsheet, print off and have it on a clipboard under your pillow. Just make sure that you click the pen cap on properly when you have finished ticking all the boxes. Don't overthink it, if you lie awake wondering whether you aired the pillows for long enough then perhaps you need to focus on the Mental Health section in this book.

# EARTHING SHEETS: WHAT IS GROUNDING?

As our bodies have electromagnetic frequencies it is believed that coming into contact with the Earth's surface allows for the transfer of negatively charged electrons (5). Apparently this can reduce inflammation, stress, improve sleep, relieve pain and boost our immune systems. However, there is very limited scientific evidence to support the health claims of those who advocate grounding, or the use of earthing sheets.

Our feet have come a long way from walking barefoot through the grass, with barriers of rubber and concrete preventing a connection with the earth that we once had. The fact that the grounding advocates are very vocal about the benefits is worthy of note.

**What the sheets claim to do:**

An earthing sheet is basically a sheet with copper or silver woven into it with a thin cable that plugs into an electric socket. The plug is only connected to the earthing system of your home so there is no electrical usage nor risk. They can be kept plugged in 24/7 and only disconnected to wash, which can be laundered in your home machine.

The potential health benefits are that they can improve sleep quality, enabling the user to awake significantly refreshed, rested and energised. It is advised to have as much direct skin contact as possible with the earthing sheet. There are bold claims of reducing inflammation, relieving pain and improving circulation and energy levels, plus a reduction in anxiety, migraines and panic attacks. However, this could be argued that if one was sleeping better then such benefits would be achieved by default, so I had to try one.

I bought my earthing sheet being somewhat sceptical, as I didn't really want it to work. When the sheet arrived I put it lengthways on my bed and used paracord to hold it in place around the mattress. The cord was uncomfortable around my hands under the pillow and around my feet. I persevered for too long before I simply lay it sideways onto the bed and tucked it in! Granted it doesn't cover the whole of me but it still does the job. Through the passing of time I'll invest in a king-size one that I can tuck in.

I wanted to say that earthing sheets are just woo-woo nonsense, but I have to say that my sleep has been much deeper in recent months, and I do awake feeling more refreshed. Since using the sheet I have even woken up groggy from quality deep or REM sleep instead of my usual waking up from a light sleep and being ready to go. I guess I needed it. An earthing sheet is certainly part of my sleep arsenal from now on.

An earthing sheet advert pinged up on Facebook recently and I read some of the comments which seemed very polarised. Many people were singing the sheets praises, claiming all sorts of slumber success stories, yet the ones who were jeering at them as being bogus had one single common denominator: they hadn't actually tried the sheets for themselves, they just mocked those who had. So there you have it, bogus or a boon, silly or soporific; the reality with earthing sheets is that you'll simply have to try one out for yourself.

# FLOOR

No sleep book should be without a section on sleeping on the floor, but many people ignore this phenomenon, as it is, frankly, rare in Western society. It is true to say that our modern furniture makes us weak. All the support provided in sofas, comfy chairs and beds has taken away the strength in many of our accessory muscles. Don't believe me? Try sitting cross legged on the floor for an hour (cushions allowed), or try watching a film whilst sitting/lounging on the floor, and supporting yourself with your arms. Maybe try lasting ten minutes.

All the articles suggest that sleeping on the floor may help with back pain, as opposed to a nice soft and comfy mattress. So, are mattress designers in cahoots with chiropractors? It does seem odd to think that a hard floor is better than a soft mattress for a bad back, and yet memory foam is supposed to help bad backs? Further investigation raises some interesting points.

There are so many positive review videos of floor sleeping on YouTube, and I've only watched the ones where people have done so for over a month, as a few days is not enough to be credible. Both GPs and chiropractors have advised their patients with back pain to try sleeping on the floor for a few days/weeks with astonishing success. The YouTube comments are also full of people who have tried the floor due to back pain and then not returned to a bed since, and other full-time floor sleepers who have developed new aches and pains from sleeping in a bed whilst visiting relatives, on business trips or on holidays.

One floor sleeping advocate was saying that if you go to bed all tensed up then it can be quite difficult to let that tension go, whereas on the floor if you remain tense then it will be very uncomfortable, so it forces your body to relax. Others say that by lying on your back on the floor you support your body with your skeleton, therefore allowing the muscles to relax, as opposed to being half tensed to support your frame on a mattress, particularly a soft one.

A downside to floor sleeping is that mould can accumulate under your bedding due to a lack of air circulation at floor level. There is a potential for allergy sufferers to struggle as there is more likely to be dust and dirt circulating on the floor. Being cooler on the floor is a seasonal disadvantage or advantage depending on the time of year. Most of the floor sleeping advocates complain that it is their inability to persuade their partners to try sleeping on the floor that is the main reason why they have returned to a bed, for obvious reasons.

**My experience** of sleeping on the floor was beneficial, but will I be doing this full time? The short answer is no, I won't. However, I did feel the benefits in two main ways. Firstly, when I got into my floor-bed it wasn't comfortable enough to be sitting up reading or doom-scrolling on my telephone; in fact it wasn't comfortable to be sitting up at all, so I lay down in a relaxed position straightaway, and the lack of stimuli enabled me to switch my mind off sooner as well.

The second advantage was that I really was building and strengthening my smaller supporting muscles, tendons etc. I did wake up aching a bit, but it was the ache of gentle exercise, not the ache of a bad back/killer workout, so I knew that my body was being strengthened. I did manage a full week, but the problem was that I was also staying at friends and relatives, so I wasn't in my usual surroundings the whole time. Plus, I consumed a little too much alcohol whilst staying up chatting, so it wasn't exactly a fair trial, and I was glad to get home and return to my own bed.

I don't feel that I have any more to prove, and I don't want to get to like it too much and therefore become so familiar with floor sleeping that it becomes an issue for when I share my life with someone.

Better for me to keep things ticking along in a regular bed and have such a conversation to try floor sleeping together and go from there. Unless the waterbed's a winner.

**Final point**, if you do have a bad back, and nothing else seems to work, then try sleeping on the floor for one night. It won't kill you, even if your sleep wasn't great, and you might find that the pain has eased a little. Keep at it for a few days and see how you go.

## HAMMOCK

Seriously? Moving on from the floor to the air, hammocks also seem to have a cult following, but this really is a niche market. There seem to be two main methods of fixing the hammock; firstly, by fixing some form of plate with a U bolt on it to the walls to hook the ropes through at each end. The other is to buy a hammock stand and have it free standing in your home. Don't be put off using the wall if you rent, as you can always fill, sand and overpaint where the holes were when you leave, with door frames and behind curtains being more hidden areas of fixing. If in doubt, ask advice from a friend, as you really need to ensure a solid wall fixing. You could always fix a piece of wood to the wall and screw your fixing into the wood.

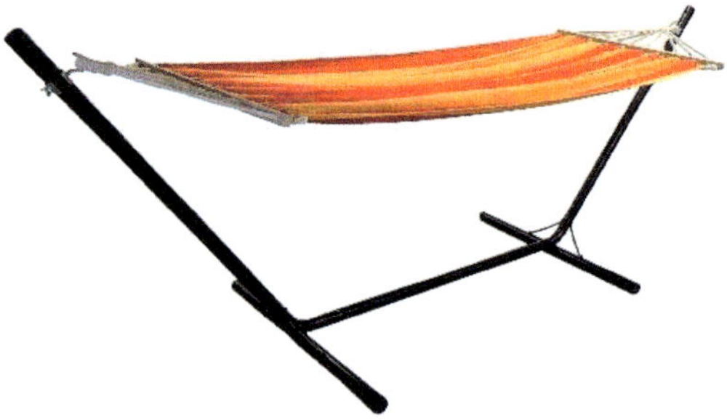

The main advantages most frequently mentioned are a reduction in back pain, a better night's sleep and they are easy to keep clean and tidy. People say that you can fall asleep more quickly, and sleep more deeply due the swinging motion of the hammock. You don't need a pillow, but some form of head/neck support may be welcomed. They are also quite relaxing for chilling or taking naps during the day, and swinging in a hammock may help reduce anxiety and have a calming effect. They are considered to be a great stress reliever. Pictured is an entry-level hammock and stand for £39.99 on Amazon. If you have a room big enough then you can start with naps before spending a whole night on one. Chilling on a hammock with a book beats slobbing on a sofa watching TV.

They are also the minimalist's dream, and are a relatively cheap option considering the average price of a bed and mattress, plus they are hypoallergenic as dust mites and bed bugs would have a hard time settling there as it is easy to launder. Regarding height, I would set it high enough to be at groin height when straddling it, it should then sag down to about 18 inches when you're settled in it. Any lower and you risk your bottom being on the floor as the new ropes adjust to having weight in them. If you need a stepladder to get in it the good luck with bathroom breaks and don't roll out, as it'll be a long way down!

Sleeping in a hammock, much like the floor, gets rave reviews from people who actually do it, but also seems to have the two same hidden dangers. Firstly, once the body gets used to it then sleeping on a normal bed usually ends up with a poor night's sleep. Secondly, and more so than the floor, hammocks are not great for intimacy, as whilst the sex on or in a hammock could be fantastic (and I'll leave that to your imagination) post-coital cuddling poses more of a challenge. Just bear in mind your combined weight if using a budget frame. Sharing is caring, but good luck having you AND your partner in the same hammock and both getting a decent night's sleep.

There are many who swear by hammocks, so if you can, give one a try. They are a pretty cool place to chill out on, and can make a nice feature and/or talking point in your home. Just try it out for naps to see how you get on before going the whole night on one. I quite like reading in mine, as my arms get nicely tucked into a good reading position, with a cushion on my lap to support the book. I'm in the perfect place for a nap too, but as I'm a side sleeper they don't work for me for a whole night.

It was hard to find books in the library on hammocks or floor sleeping and Google can be a bit hit and miss with opinions. I therefore opted for YouTube where I heard stories of real people's experiences who had actually used these alternative sleeping methods, and the comments sections on both floor and hammocks heartily agreed that each method was so much better than a regular bed. Would twin hammocks side-by-side in a modern bedroom work for you? If so, great, I'm happy for you, but for most people this notion is all at sea.

# CHAPTER 2
# BEDROOM ENVIRONMENT

## LIGHTING

Over the last few decades we have had a rapid increase in electronics, creating a technology revolution. Thanks to the internet, 24/7 shopping is now available. This means that we now have 24/7 light, and the blurring of work and leisure, with many people doing social things on their phones at work, and work things at home. Gone is the natural dimming of light with the seasons, and the sheer vastness and diversity of entertainment creates a Fear of Missing Out (FOMO) so lots of people feel the need to cram in as much as possible.

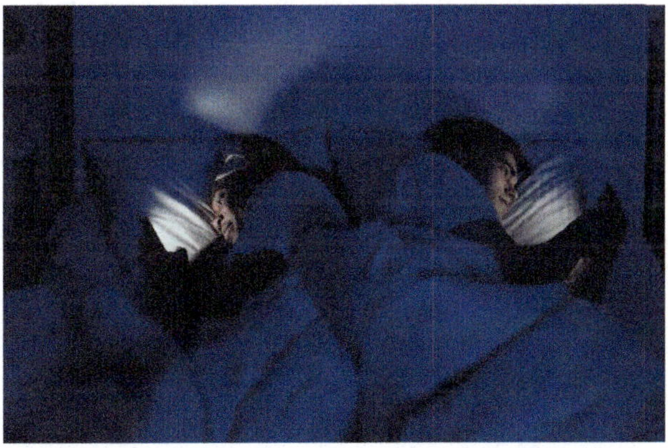

**Blue light**, or blue wavelengths are beneficial during daylight hours because they boost attention, mood and reaction times, but for this reason, they tend to be the most disruptive at night. The proliferation of electronics with screens, as well as energy-efficient lighting, is increasing our exposure to blue wavelengths, especially after sundown. Fluorescent lightbulbs and LED lights are much more energy-efficient, but they also produce more blue light than the old-fashioned incandescent lightbulbs. Dr. Charles Czeisler of Harvard Medical School showed, in 1981, that daylight keeps a person's internal clock aligned with the environment. This seems obvious but there are a surprising number of people who don't give this a second thought. Use candles and salt lamps for a soft evening glow as they help the mind wind down and are very flattering for the body.

Telephones: There are plenty of apps to download that will reduce the blue light, but they seem to do this by masking the blue light rather than removing it. I've just downloaded a free app called 'Twilight' and it seems to do the job and give the screen a red hue which I have to say is more relaxing for my eyes. However, because I don't have my location on unless using my phone as a satnav I have to press the 'approximate location' each time I switch my phone on if I want the app to run. Still, that's the trade-off with the app, but for longer phone sessions it's worth it.

F.lux is a computer program that adjusts a display's colour temperature according to your location and the time of day, as it offers functional respite for the eyes. Therefore, naturally dimming your laptop screen as dusk settles. The program is designed to reduce eye strain during night-time use, helping to reduce disruption of sleep patterns.

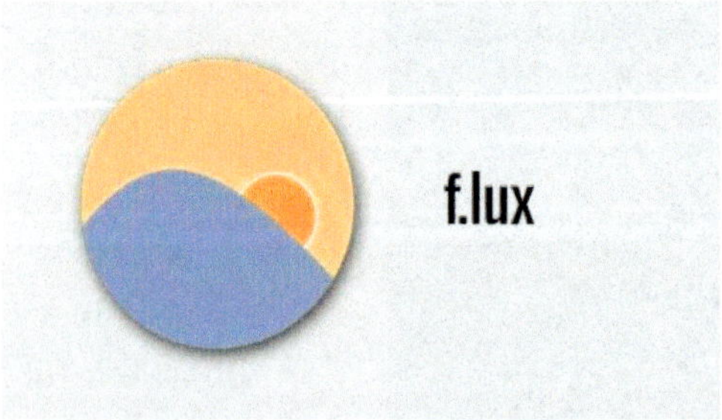


F.lux is free to install and use. This really helps my eyes when I am typing, whether during the daylight hours or in the evening. However, the brightness settings on my laptop are generally less than a quarter full every day.

I've also put a piece of black tape over the light for the smoke detectors to prevent any visual disturbance once asleep. On some models you can lift the cover off first to apply the tape to make the outside look better. It's a bit OCD, but that flashing light triggered me enough to start my mind racing and overthinking it, so the tape works for me.

# SUNLIGHT

Tonight's sleep will start from the moment that you are awake. A bold statement, but sunlight, particularly in the morning will help to regulate your circadian rhythm, which has a beneficial knock-on effect to tonight's sleep. And vice-versa.

Experts suggest 20-30 minutes of sunlight each day will help with setting your circadian rhythm (6) and may help counteract the effect of screen time during the evening. But what does this really mean? That we can tell our employer that we are just nipping outside for half an hour to remain productive today and for the rest of the week? The impracticality of this for many people is self-explanatory, so what can we do?

If you can get outside for a minute or two, just take in the fresh smell of the outside (there are always variables, I know) and enjoy the sun on your face. If you can't achieve this then try looking out of the window as much as possible particularly when you can't get out and are moving about within the building. Taking that moment to appreciate the little things and the little moments can break up your day and have a positive impact on your life. Those little moments may also help reduce stress levels, or they can get you fired if you're not discreet, so find a helpful balance.

**Blackout curtains** are a great choice for shift workers and anyone with trouble sleeping, or those wanting to recreate The Blitz.

Blackout blinds are also good, but be aware that if you buy one and fit it you'll be lucky for it to block out all the light, with the top and sides being where the light shines in the most. In my nightshift heyday I used to have a navy towel that I trapped in the sash window before drawing the curtains, and the combination together worked perfectly.

One room that I rented had no curtains at all, so I bought heavy duty lining paper and cut it to the size of the glass and taped it on. Less than ideal, but it did work. Get creative, remember that nail/screw holes can be filled before you leave, so don't let rented affect your ability to modify the windows to make covers that work for you. Thick dustsheets are also good for larger windows, use hooks and poke a hole in the dustsheet. I get that it may not be aesthetically pleasing, but for short-term function to get you through a bad patch it can be a lifesaver.

## VENTILATION

We all know that fresh air is good for us, and the bedroom is no exception. The trouble is that most of us who have had trouble sleeping at some point are generally sensitive to noise or disturbances. Unless you live in a log cabin somewhere then sleeping with the windows open post-nightshift is a non-starter. Traffic, deliveries, dogs barking, children screaming, babies crying, roadworks, someone drilling, the list is endless.

That said, even at night in more urban areas there are still traffic noises, some bonehead with his max-power car and bean-can exhaust, scooter deliveries, plus the risk of cats fighting, dogs barking and foxes making strange and scary noises. In the country there is still a risk of bats flying in through the window (happened to my brother in his teens, and landed on his pillow! He wasn't fazed, just scooped it up and popped it back outside). There are also mosquitos, daddy-long-legs (the cranefly, not the spider), midges, moths and if you're unlucky, May bugs (AKA cockchafers, which sounds painful, so I'll stick with May bugs). Internet research is a minefield of conflicting information about whether the windows should be open or closed at night, but closed windows day or night are a quieter option, and would allow more uninterrupted sleep. Just crank them open in the morning to freshen the room.

## **MOULD**

Stachybotrys chartarum AKA black mould seems to grow pretty much anywhere, favouring damp areas due to water damage, leaks, condensation and high humidity areas. It seems particularly keen on bathrooms, notably ceilings and other hard-to-reach areas. Thanks to the current winter energy price crisis in the UK, it has crept into bedrooms and other areas that either cannot afford to be heated, or are naturally damp, or both. One of the best mould preventions is adequate heating and opening windows to allow the free-flow or air; my yearly winter conundrum of keeping heat in yet providing adequate ventilation.

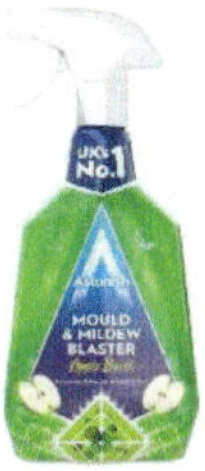


Unfortunately, the spores are almost everywhere, but thankfully it can be killed, or at least controlled, using standard household bleach.

As well as bleach, I've had good results with 'Astonish Mould and Mildew Blaster'. It really is worth tackling black mould to get rid of it, as it's not good for your respiratory health, and those prone to allergies are likely to be affected more significantly. Finally, be aware when you move home, that if your furniture has black mould on it then you could be taking it with you to your new place.

## TEMPERATURE

Having trawled through endless sleep books to attempt to find a gold standard, the general concensus is that between 60-68 degrees Fahrenheit or about 16-20 degrees Celsius is the best temperature to sleep in. Obviously this is going to vary from person to person, so adjust accordingly. I have to agree, having slept in a range of temperatures here in the UK from about 5C/40F degrees in the winter to about 27C/80F in the summer (both inside), I have to say that a balmy 18C/65F sounds delightful. For obvious reasons I sleep better in the spring and autumn.

## WHEN IT'S TOO HOT

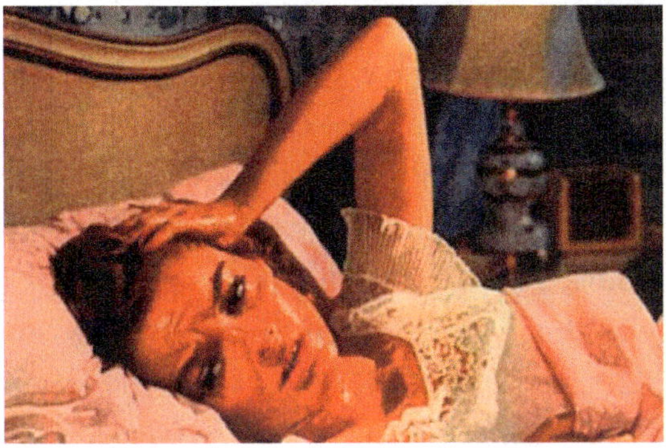

Sleeping in a room that is too hot can cause more frequent awakenings throughout the night, excessive sweating, and the disruption of REM (Rapid Eye Movement) sleep. Who'd have thought? But you've not got any more clothes to take off, so what do you do? Use cold flannels, ice cubes in a plastic bag or that old bag of frozen peas from Kwik-Save that you keep for sprained ankles and twisted knees (just stick them inside a pillow case for comfort on your skin) and you'll be amazed at how quickly you can cool down. Try a hot water bottle filled with ice cubes and cold water; works a treat. Or put a wet flannel in the freezer just before bed and it'll be lovely and cold to reduce your body temperature. You could also take a couple of paracetamol (or just one if you're under 50kg) and that'll reduce your temperature for at least 3-4 hours too. Lukewarm showers take a bit more effort, and cold ones considerably more, but you'll be hot again soon enough so just get on with it. Or, run your hands and wrists under the cold tap as it's a quick and easy way to reduce your temperature. A bucket of cold water by your chamber pot to dunk your feet in can really help when you're sweating away at 2am, just don't forget a towel; and get the right bucket.

Limit or avoid alcohol, as processing it will heat up your body, and dehydrate you. Ditto a high protein intake, as it heightens your metabolic rate in a similar way. If you can sleep alone then try to; at least you'll both sleep better, knowing that you're not lying next to a furnace! That way you can stretch out, which is also very cooling, due to the greater surface area exposed to the bed.

In the summertime, it can be better to leave windows and curtains closed during the day as they can let in extra heat making your bedroom too hot to sleep at night. Don't bother buying a cheap supermarket fan. They'll be noisy, creaky as they oscillate and basically blow the warm air all around the room, scattering dust as they go. A Dyson Purifier Cool removes 99.5% of the airborne pollutants, including formaldehyde found in carpets and floors as well as the usual bacteria and allergens. It also cools the room.

## WHEN IT'S TOO COLD

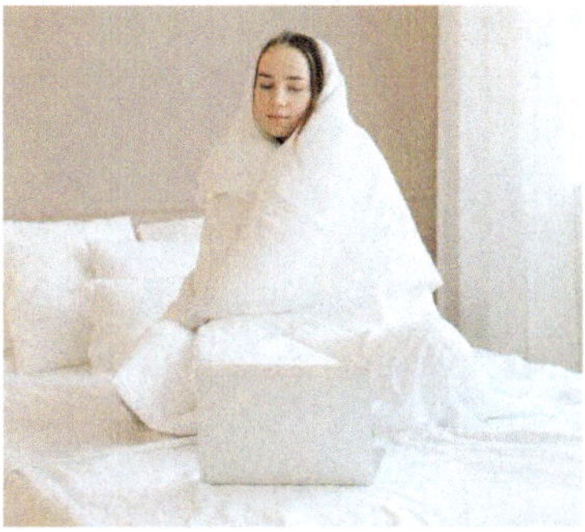

Apparently there is a risk of inflammation of the lungs, inhibited circulation and an increase in respiratory conditions; also, one may be more susceptible to bacterial or viral infections and depression by sleeping in a room that is too cold. Great. However, the misery of being too cold can be combatted by wearing more clothes, woolly hats, electric blankets and hot-water bottles. Or basically do the opposite of what you'd do if you are too hot.

Just bear in mind when you're complaining about the temperature that our Inuit and African cousins sleep in extreme temperatures and are healthy enough, as do people in mid-Europe where temperatures soar and plummet with the seasons (Hungary ranges from -10C/17F to 35C/95F degrees. This may not really help you, but it is true to say that there is always someone worse off than you are who just gets on with it.

# CHAPTER 3
# INTIMACY

Sleeping without any clothes on is actually good for your health. Allowing air to get to your body parts that are usually covered up during the day is beneficial. Think of feet, armpits and groins; by being unclothed overnight the delicate skin around all these areas can breathe, reducing the risk of potential fungal infections developing. Of this I shall elaborate no more, but it is applicable for both men and for women. For men, allowing the testes freedom from underwear provides better thermoregulation, resulting a higher sperm count. If groins are landscaped then this reduces the risk of ingrowing hairs or rashes. Sleeping naked also helps with fat loss, as the body will be naturally cooler and therefore burn fat for warmth as you sleep. It's not exactly a diet pill, but every little helps.

Oxytocin is a hormone that is typically linked to pair bonding among humans and it helps to create warm, fuzzy feelings (7). It is shown in some research to lower stress levels and anxiety. Oxytocin has the power to regulate our emotional responses and behaviours, including trust, empathy, gazing and positive memories. Skin to skin contact, even without a sexual connotation, gets the love chemical flowing. This could be a reason why mothers tend to bond closer with their children, due to more skin-to-skin contact from an early age, often during breastfeeding and bathing. Couples who let this oxytocin chemical flow freely together often have stronger and longer relationships. It makes sense that couples who get naked and cuddle have stronger relationships, but any cuddling is beneficial, naked or clothed.

According to a University of Arizona study, adults who share a bed with a partner sleep better than those who sleep alone (8). Personally, I really struggle with this statement, perhaps because of my own unique experience of my long-forgotten past, or perhaps because I've worked with so many people who have complained about their respective partners being such unpleasant people, that the whole idea of sleeping better together is an urban myth. If it's true, and if it works for you then fantastic, I'm genuinely happy for you. Researchers suggest that sleeping with a partner decreases anxiety and increases relationship connection, and that the oxytocin released can help people wake up more refreshed. Apparently.

However, not all of us are comfortable sleeping naked, so what are the alternatives for a good night's sleep? The history of bedclothes dates back a very long way, but I shall be focussing on function rather than fashion. What you choose to wear or not wear is up to you, and here it remains private to how anyone chooses to express their sexuality with their nightclothes.

**Nightgowns** were traditionally worn by both men and women. Nightgowns for women had the name shorted to 'nighty' in the 1920's, which was also the time that negligees came into fashion, with many designed to mimic the flapper-style clothing that was popular at the time. Look up 'Cottagecore' to find a whole range of traditional nightwear and clothing. Like most modern clothing, as time went on, shorter and sexier styles were developed. This is as erotic as I shall go regarding women's nightwear.

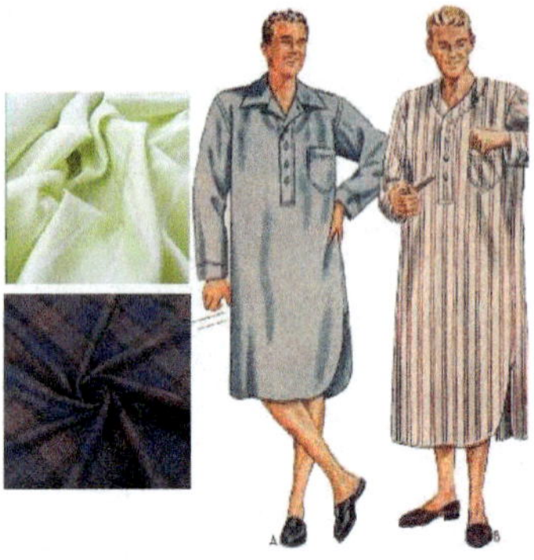

Men's nightgowns generally look like an elongated shirt, down to the knees. This type of tunic has been around for thousands of years, and has changed little. Think of Dickens' character of Ebenezer Scrooge wandering along cold corridors at night with his candle-stick looking for ghosties or a midnight snack. Is it fair to label a nightgown as *old man's apparel?* Well, they certainly allowed for range of movement for those with restless legs, and allowed for suitable circulation for the groin area, so why did they go out of fashion for men? Enter the pyjama phase…

**Pyjamas** replaced men's nightgowns from around the 1870s by British men who were returning from India in the $18^{th}$ and $19^{th}$ centuries. In Hindi the term 'pae jama' or 'pai jama' literally translates as 'garment for the legs'. However, they didn't become popular until the 1920s when fashion was changing and new options were becoming available. Cotton and silk were the general fabric choices, and different colours and cuts were made available for everyday people. PJs were initially made with long sleeves and had full-length legs, with shorter versions becoming more common later.

Pyjamas for women also entered the sleepwear scene during the 1920s, and became a form of evening loungewear post World War 1 as attitudes relaxed and women became more prominent in society.

Men's modern lounge sets are generally made from cotton or a cotton/polyester blend. They tend to be more comfortable than the traditional cotton 'stripey' PJs as they are more stretchy and therefore more comfortable for the fidgety sleeper. I've had some terribly restricted night's sleep in traditional style cotton PJs and some great nights' sleep in modern loungewear.

**Shorts** are a viable option, favoured by military, police and other service chaps as they enable the wearer to leap out of bed and protect the household contents or vehicles without even having to think of donning clothes. A real get up and go attitude, but it could save lives and I guess it's good to be prepared. Pyjama shorts would be a better choice being purpose built for sleeping, with more comfortable and breathable fabric.

**Boxer shorts** are favoured by many men, but a word of caution is required. Some modern boxers have Lycra/polyester in them. That and the general tightness of boxer/briefs do not allow for good jewel health. The all-cotton traditional style can really get caught up whilst you sleep, and this area of the body requires good circulation. Many a night of my youth has been with poor sleep due to this problem, much like when you cross your legs and your testicles wish that you hadn't. The body puts up a protest, you wake up, drag the fabric down, dab your eyes and then find yourself tossing and turning for hours. Re-read the paragraph about the benefits of sleeping naked or choose your garments wisely.

**Onesies** sadly have to get a mention. If you had a childhood dream to look like Andy Pandy or one of the Teletubbies then they could be just for you. However, on a practical note, I can't imagine the trauma of having to let all that heat out in wintertime for a 2am lavatory break. Okay, so for the chaps I have discovered that there are two-way zippers, so that's the standing problem sorted. However, I am dismayed to discover that there are onesies with a flap at the back for seated toileting. Yuck. There are also websites that advise on how to pee whilst wearing a onesie, so have a look, if you must.

## SEX & SEXUALITY

No sleep book could be complete without acknowledging sex and sexuality. As adult humans, we are sexual beings whether we like to admit it or not. However, most of us will know that an orgasm will provide the body with some form of release and indeed, relief. This can be beneficial in resetting and relaxing the body before sleep, it can also be addictive, and create dependency, whether alone or with your partner. Whatever you do will hopefully remain personal to you.

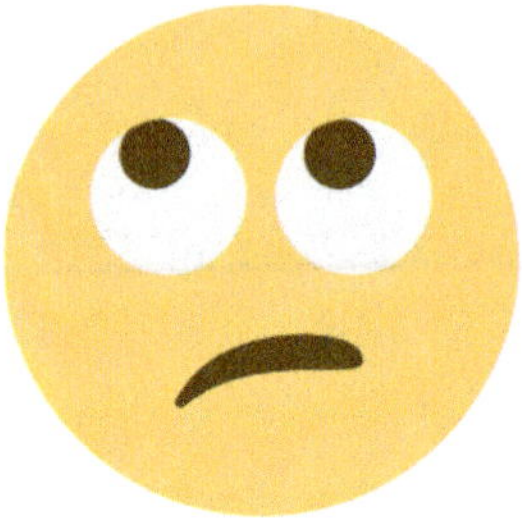

Some may be disappointed that such an interesting and emotive subject is being glossed over, others may be quite relieved. What I do know is that sex is a private matter, and should be kept as such.

## PETS OR PESTS?

Most of us love animals, and many of us like to have them in our homes, as a pet. Some people even allow their animals into their bedroom, and apparently, even onto their beds. If this works for you then great, I'm happy for you. However, cats and dogs leave dust, dander and allergens that can cause breathing problems that can potentially disrupt your slumber. Pets moving around on the bed or in the bedroom may be waking you up without you realising that it's them.

A good night's sleep is a fair price to pay for putting Kitty or Doggo into the kitchen, as you don't want them scratching at the door or jumping on your bed at an unearthly hour. Even a fish tank can disrupt sleep, with the lights, pump noise, bubbles, etc. Your pet may provide great comfort for you, and that is really very wonderful, but they could also be the elephant in your room.

## CHILDREN

Allowing your children to sleep in your bed can be lovely, but usually only for the child. It always seemed like a bad idea to me, so I had this conversation with my children's mother at the relevant time, and we agreed that after about 6 weeks the baby was to go into their own room. That way, neither of our children ever got a feel for sleeping in our bed so that there would not come a day when they would insanely protest against their room transfer.

It is a good idea to talk with your partner to establish some housekeeping rules about sleeping with children in your bed *before* they arrive. Well, you do live together, so it is far better to discuss and negotiate routines and preferences rather than just letting things pan out as they do. You may find that you end up tolerating way too much, and vice-versa.

I can honestly say that I have never actually shared a night with either of my children in our bed, and they are teenagers now, so never will. I have heard stories of the horrendous struggle that parents have had to get their child out of their bed and into the child's own bed. You make a rod for your own back; every action has a reaction, and all that. Before I am labelled as completely heartless we did practise 'controlled crying' whereby we'd settle our children down, say goodnight and leave the room, and then return in about 1-2 minutes to reassure our child, then leave, then increase the time away from our child and keep repeating until they self-settled and slept.

I remember one night where we were both so tired and one of them had woken up past midnight and we were doing the whole tag-team of settling them down and their mother cracked and suggested that we just kept him/her in our bed for a few hours so that we can all sleep but I declined to acquiesce and stuck with the program. One night of sabotaged sleep is better than weeks or months of ongoing headaches from a child who demands to sleep in our bed again. My child settled shortly afterwards after what seemed like hours and the rest is history. If it works for you having a child in your bed then great, I'm happy for you all, but if it doesn't then sit down and talk about how to make an extraction plan. It will benefit you all in the long run.

## SLEEP POSITIONS

## IS THERE REALLY A CORRECT POSITION TO SLEEP IN?

Research suggests that most people prefer to sleep in the foetal position, on their sides (9). Sleep experts have also discovered that people who sleep in the supine position (on their backs - think 'spine' and 'back') usually have a poorer quality of sleep and often experience breathing difficulties. Anyone who has been around people who snore would likely agree with this.

In the same study they demonstrated that of the 664 sleepers, the average participants spent about 54.1 percent of their time sleeping on their side, about 37.5 percent on their back, and about 7.3 percent on their front. They never accounted for the other 1.1 percent, but that's statistics for you. In most cases, we tend to move around quite a lot during the night, with males (especially those aged under 35) tending to be most restless.

This is actually a good thing, because by allowing your body to move about during the night keeps the circulation going and will prevent pressure ulcers (bedsores) from developing on your bony prominences (think lower back, heels, shoulder blades to name a few). Ever gone to bed with a stiff neck and woken up pain-free? Chances are your body moved into an uncomfortable position whilst asleep and 'stretched-out' the muscles causing the pain. Beware of tucking in the bedsheets too tightly. See the previous bedding section for reasons why. This includes untucking hotel bed sheets to allow your feet to have freedom of movement overnight. 'But it looks untidy in my nice hotel room!' Maybe so, but for a good night's sleep it can be a fair compromise.

The correct position to sleep in is one that works for YOU. There are so many factors such as your environment, age, weight, etc., so find what works to avoid pain and provide rest and the best sleep that you can get. Bear in mind that sleeping on your side may cause some form of spinal rotation which can cause pain upon waking, but sleeping in the prone position (on your front) or supine carry their own set of problems, so side-sleeping is generally to be favoured.

## SNORING

Snoring usually occurs due to the vibration of the tissues in the throat (10). It is the result of turbulent airflow and vibrations in the soft tissues of the upper airway, says Kevin Motz, MD, assistant professor of otolaryngology (general ENT stuff) and director of sleep surgery at Johns Hopkins Medicine. Snoring devices are aimed at increasing airflow, stiffening the upper airway, or reducing turbulent airflow, which occurs if the tissue has become narrow and collapsed. "These work by dilating the airway in some manner, or preventing what we call flow limitation," Dr. Motz says. For those who have suffered a poor night's sleep next to or near to someone who snores, I feel your pain. However, some people may need to be told that no-one goes to bed and plans to snore. It is what it is.

Snoring can be comparable to those who flatulate whilst asleep (I try to avoid the term *farting*). It remains unplanned, and well, just happens. Whilst dietary habits can, to a degree, reduce the desire to flirt with flatulence, they can also be considered to avoid excessive snoring. This is particularly true for alcohol consumption. In the not-so-distant past I have, whilst visiting relatives, consumed too much red wine, and it has been reported back to me that upon retiring to bed I fell asleep almost instantly and snored like Billy-o. Whoops, sorry folks.

There is also a direct corroboration between being overweight and snoring. The Mayo Clinic, and many others have extensive research do conclude what we all hopefully knew as common sense; the more weight one carries, the more adipose tissue will fill compartments (the soft tissues in respiratory areas) causing restrictions and inhibiting breathing. Central obesity with make breathing harder as well due to making the effort of breathing more constricted. All this, in case unknown, is likely to contribute to snoring, so there really is something that can be done: lose weight. Easier said than done, but this is a sleep book, not a diet book. However, if you make a plan, and truly want it enough, then you can set your face like flint to achieve your goal. But you've got to want it enough…

## SEPTOPLASTY/RHINOPLASTY

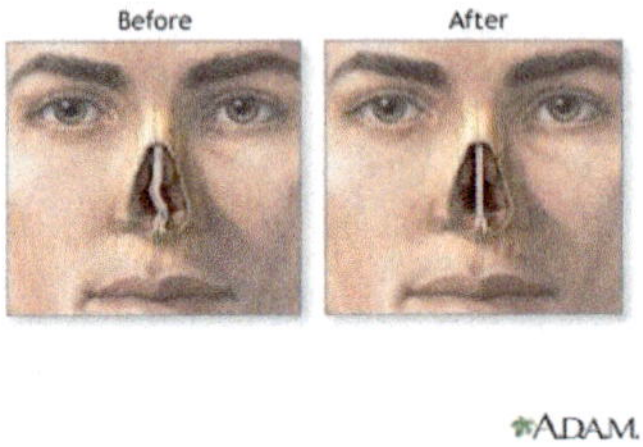


The septum is the middle bit of tissue that separates the nostrils. This picture clearly demonstrates a deviated septum on the left, and after surgery (or before injury) on the right (11). Thanks to a class bully I got my nose broken as a teenager but it wasn't until I slept next to someone (my then wife after getting married) that she informed me what a poor sleeper that I was. I simply assumed that feeling so tired every day was part of the aging process (seriously, I did, and I was only 25!) and me being a self-confessed 'poor sleeper' (which is a very bad thing to declare over yourself). A trip to the GP ensued an ENT referral and the rest is history. I was a student nurse at the time, and for the record, I went back into college post-op day one the very next morning. I felt hammered (literally, from the op) and still groggy from the anaesthesia so I walked as I couldn't risk cycle in. I figured that when qualified, I'd be telling my patients that they need to try to recuperate and get things back to normal, so I had to walk the walk. In class I couldn't concentrate on anything, watery snot and blood were leaking from my nose and my face was so swollen that they sent me home at lunchtime, but I did try. I would therefore advise others to rest post-op day one. To conclude, when I could breathe again, it was marvellous. Not the panacea of all my sleeping woes but I seemed to have more energy from breathing and sleeping better. I was a bit miffed that the surgeon only did the septoplasty and didn't include a rhinoplasty as well, so my nose remains slightly wonky, but that's life.

For those who can afford it, the excuse of snoring and a deviated septum could be just the excuse for getting a nose-job done, but be careful, cosmetic surgery can become addictive. Thankfully I've worked on my inner junk so I am far less concerned about my outer shell, so try that for yourself first; it's far cheaper and you'll probably find yourself happier in the long run anyway. That said, the septoplasty worked very well for me.

Here are some simple devices that are available to help prevent snoring, and for the cost they are probably worth a go.

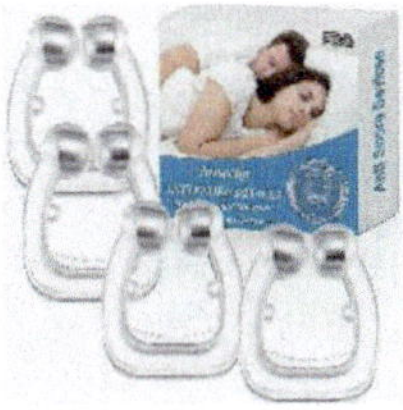

Stick this device up your nostrils to open the airway and prevent snoring.

Less than £5 on eBay.

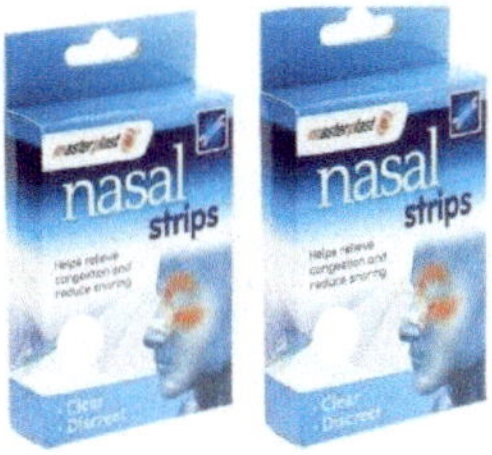


Use these strips on the bridge of your nose like some marathon runners do. Definitely help with breathing, may not help with snoring. Try Steri-Strips at a pinch. Less than £5 on eBay.

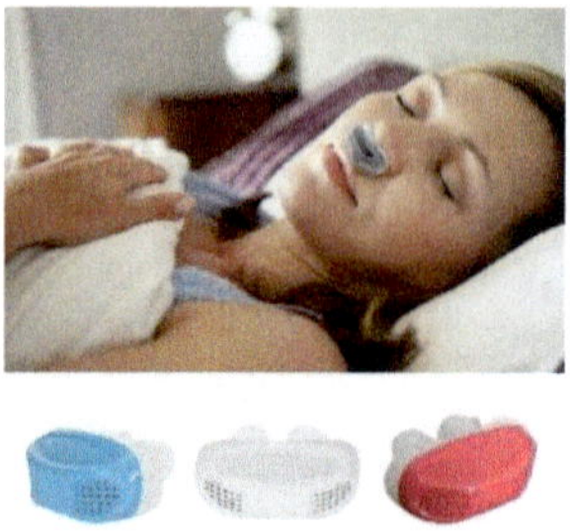

This device has a unique aesthetic about it; it looks gross. Available for less than £5 on eBay.

Excitingly there is another model that can be charged up via USB and has a mini-fan to gently blow air up your nostrils as you drift off. Sounds magnificent, and is available for less than £10 on eBay.

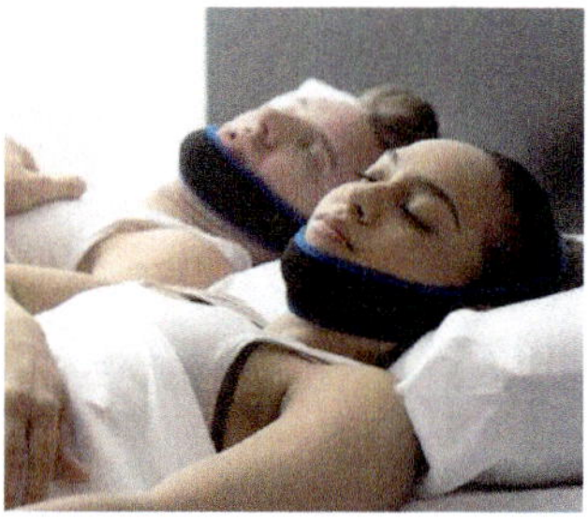

So sleeping with your mouth open can cause snoring. Who would have thought that? Here we have an 'anti-snoring aid' that solves the problem at source; by keeping your mouth closed overnight.

Another less than £5 masterpiece from eBay. It might actually feel quite reassuring and comforting having that in place, it would certainly help prevent drooling whilst asleep.

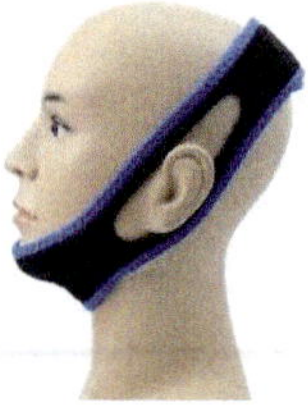

However, judging by the vacant stare on the model's face, this one seems like a bit of a wild card.

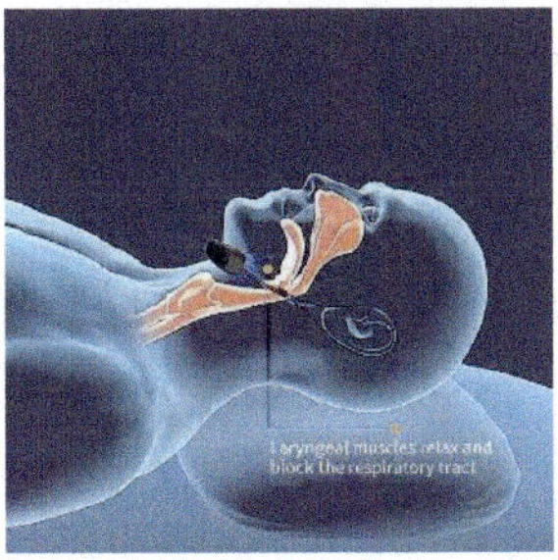


Similar to the one above, this product will automatically and accurately detect the snoring sound through high-precision sensors, and massage the hypoglossal nerve and mandibular muscles through vibration pulses of different frequencies to promote muscle tightening, adjust the breathing rhythm, and make breathing smoother; less than £10 on eBay.

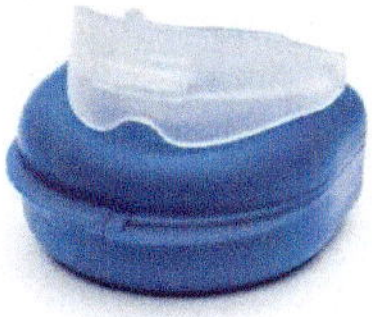

Fitting like a boxer's gumshield, this 'boil & bite' mouthguard costs less than £10.

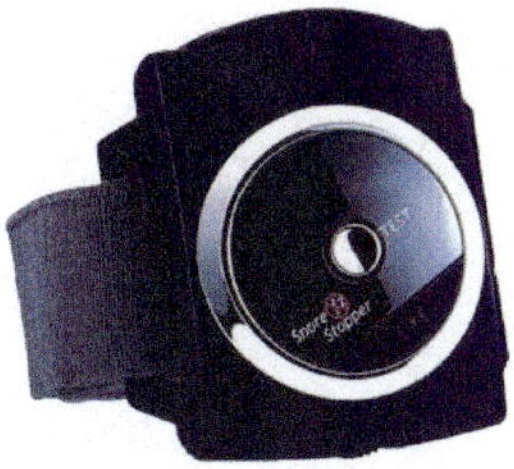


Electronic Snore Stopper.

Emits a micro-pulse like a nudge; less than £10 on eBay.

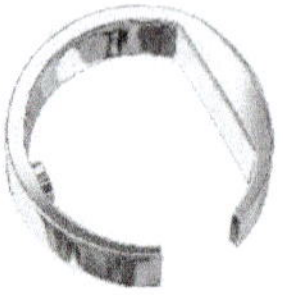

Apparently this ring is supposed to stop snoring by using magnets and acupressure to dilate your breathing. Worn on the little finger about 30 minutes before bed, it is a fairly unintrusive method, and I'm reluctant to poo-poo said ring as it may just work. The Oura sleep ring has a similar bumps on the inside which makes this ring appear more credible. For under £10 I'd give it a go.

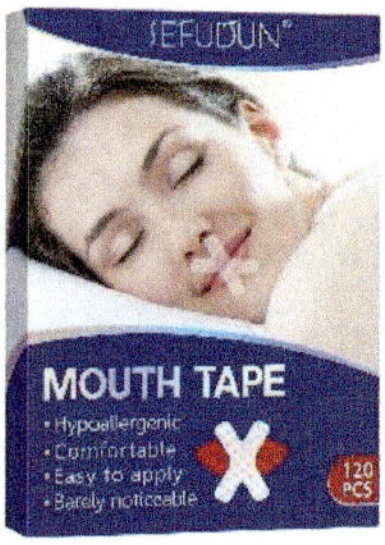


Finally, what stop-snoring accessory guide would be complete without providing details about mouth tape? Yes, you really can buy it from Amazon and people do use it. So, if all else fails and you're fed up with your partners snoring then at least you can tape their mouth shut!

# SPIDER BREATH?

Do we really swallow up to eight spiders per year whilst we are asleep? I thought that the easiest place to discover if this is true would be on the web. Most of us do indeed, sleep with our mouths closed. However, if our mouths are open then we may well be snoring, but if not, our breathing will send powerful vibrations out of our mouth and lips. Spiders are fine tuned to vibrations, hence why when a fly lands on their web they are straight out for the kill, and why trapdoor spiders can remain out of sight as they feel the vibrations of their prey.

This is great news for us, as all the research suggests that it is extremely unlikely for a spider to crawl into a sleeping person's mouth, as our breathing vibrations will scare the spider away. Some twenty years ago I was joking with other student nurses about why our morning breath was so foul as a possibility of being due to the spider that we ate during our sleep. Spider breath? However, having extensively trawled the web for articles, testimonials or video proof, no evidence has materialised that could confirm such a nocturnal arachnid feast has ever occurred, so myth busted. You could always be the first though. Tonight. Cue the creepy laugh…!

# CHAPTER 4
# SLEEP STAGES AND SLEEP CYCLES

Experts say that our sleep stages really do matter (and they do). You don't need to be told that a healthy sleep cycle is an important factor in your overall health. Go too long without sleep and your body will soon protest. Studies have shown a connection between sleep deprivation and weight gain, and being a cause of acne in women. Many people believe that the brain "shuts off" during sleep to enable it to rest. However, this is not necessarily the case, as there is more going on whilst asleep that we may think. The brain goes through several different cycles throughout the time that we are sleeping.

These cycles change throughout the different stages of sleep, starting with NREM (Non-Rapid Eye Movement) sleep and progressing to the REM (Rapid Eye Movement) sleep. The typical person starts a new sleep cycle every 90 to 120 minutes, meaning they likely go through four or five cycles during a night of rest (12).

Here we'll cover the different stages of sleep, which are the most important, how much sleep we should get and how sleep changes throughout a lifetime.

| STAGE 1 | STAGE 2 | STAGE 3 | STAGE 4 |
|---|---|---|---|
| NREM SLEEP<br><br>2-5% | NREM SLEEP<br><br>45-55% | NREM SLEEP<br><br>13-23% | REM SLEEP<br><br>20-25% |
| 5-10 MINUTES | 4-7 HOURS PER NIGHT | DEEP SLEEP<br><br>45-90 MINUTES | 90-120 MINUTES |

**Stage 1:** This first stage is very light, and you can be easily woken; think of someone who has nodded off whist watching a film. Your body starts to relax and you become drowsy. Your eyes may move a little, but not significantly. A gentle snore is enough to wake someone at this stage (but never you, as you don't snore do you?). Some people also experience sudden jerks or muscle spasms during this stage, known in the medical world as myoclonus (with a more common form being the hiccup).

There have been many times when I've been watching a DVD with my children and I'd not noticed that they had fallen asleep next to me (The A-Team can be quite tense) and their leg has briefly shot out and then settled whilst they've been fast asleep. Definitely happens more with children, as I'm yet to see it with elderly people in hospital or care homes, and I've seen a few, but perhaps if they watched The A-Team then they might?

During this phase your brain waves slow down as your body begins to relax. This stage lasts for about 1-10 minutes. People who wake from Stage 1 sleep often will deny being asleep, they can also wake and appear very alert and resume tasks with little change, despite being asleep. Strange and vivid sensations are known as 'hypnagogic hallucinations.' The brain activity in in an 'alpha wave' state during stage 1.

**Stage 2:** Moving on from Stage 1 happens fairly quickly, and your eyes and body settle down and become still, as your muscles relax further. Spasms are unlikely at this stage and your body goes into a standby-like state. Generally speaking, your temperature dips as you fall into a deeper sleep. Your breathing also lowers, along with your heart rate.

This is still considered a light sleep, but hopefully you're heading for a deeper stage. People who get woken up during Stage 2 sleep often feel well-rested and refreshed, and there is a danger to get up and carry on because you feel okay. Please don't, your body needs the deeper stuff. Stage 2 makes up the main body of your sleep cycle, comprising 4-7 hours per night.

**Stage 3:** This is the deep sleep stage, and is the most restorative part of the sleep cycle. Your eyes are still during this phase, and your body doesn't move about at all during the deep sleep due to being so relaxed. Your heart beats at its slowest, your blood pressure drops and your breathing is at its calmest. It is during this sleep that your body starts its physical repairs, regrowing tissue, rebuilding bones, muscles and the immune system.

Your brain, in contrast to your body, is surprisingly active during this deep stage of sleep. Experts have identified brain activity called delta waves or slow wave sleep. This is the most difficult stage to awaken from, and for some people, even loud noises greater than 100 decibels will not wake them up. Stage 3 cycles are 45-90 minutes.

**Sleep inertia** is the term given to a physiological state of impaired cognitive and motor functions, with feelings of drowsiness, mental fogginess (such as disorientation) and a decline in motor dexterity causing an inability to perform tasks very well. This experience may last from 15 minutes up to an hour. If woken during this sleep phase then the person is likely to experience grogginess and the feeling of an unsatisfied sleep. This is also the stage when sleepwalking, night terrors, and bedwetting occurs; none of which are an amusing phenomenon.

**Stage 4:** Rapid Eye Movement (REM) sleep is interesting because the brain becomes more active and yet the body becomes more lethargic. As per the name, your eyes move rapidly, your heart rate and breathing increase and your brain activity speeds up to the level of when you are awake. It is easier to wake up during REM than at stage 3, but like the deep sleep, you'll feel groggy and unrested. Most people have 3-5 REM cycles per night, which can be between 10-60 minutes.

We tend to dream more vividly during REM, hence why you remember your dreams in detail, although it is likely that you will have woken at the end of a REM cycle or mid-cycle when your alarm went off. The experts suggest that over three-quarters of your vivid dream recall results from your REM sleep. My cynical explanation for that would be that you generally tend to remember your last dream before you awoke, rather than the one that you had at midnight.

## Sleep Cycles Concluded

As with all the timings on the charts, they are just guidelines as everyone's sleep pattern is different. Factors such as waking up after a nightmare, waking to use the lavatory, telephone calls, emergencies etc., can all skew the order of the sleep cycle, or even prevent a cycle from occurring at all. Environmental and lifestyle choices can skew the cycle further, with alcohol, nicotine, caffeine, partner snoring, being overweight, breathing issues, worry and the list could go on, so your sleep patterns may not follow the simple progression of Stages 1-4.

# HOW DOES INSOMNIA AFFECT OUR HEALTH?

Global organisations such as the WHO and the Centers for Disease Control and Prevention (CDC) suggest that over a third of the USA gets less than seven hours of sleep every 24 hours (13). Perhaps all the technology that is driving us into the 'fourth industrial revolution' is keeping us permanently switched on?

I hope that everyone knows that their own lifestyle habits, such as: lack of exercise, smoking/vaping, excessive caffeine intake, excessive alcohol will, to some degree, affect their sleep as well as their overall health. However, poor sleep has been linked to other health conditions including; Alzheimer's, Parkinson's, obesity, heart disease, asthma, fibromyalgia (and other chronic pain conditions, plus auto-immune diseases), obstructive sleep apnoea and restless leg syndrome (14). Every aspect of our bodies will suffer to some degree, and our immune system can really take a hammering, making us more vulnerable to illnesses, and if you're in the UK; the dreaded lurgy.

Most people will know that a lack of sleep is not happy days, and may well affect your daily tasks as highlighted below:

- Memory recall.
- Retaining information and learning.
- Rational decision making and problem solving.
- Creativity will likely suffer.
- Self-control of your emotions and behaviours.

So, in a nutshell, when you drop something, you're more likely to stamp your feet and say 'bother' or use a stronger and more universal term. Seriously, things really bug us when we're sleep deprived.

Suffice to say that a lack thereof affects everything about us, including our quality of life, so let's get some more of it.

# HOW MUCH SLEEP DO I NEED?

The CDC, after their US study, recommend that adults get between seven and nine hours sleep per night (15), shift workers may be envious to get five or six hours, and lying there worrying that you are not getting enough is not going to help either. The good news is that the perfect number of hours sleep does vary from person to person.

It is important to know whether you are sleepy or simply just tired. This is where 'knowing thyself' is important, but too many people seem to go around in a square-eyed haze from too much screen time. To clarify, a day of hard manual labour (housework still counts) can leave you physically tired, but not necessarily sleepy. You may also be tired during the day due to physical activities and limitations, mental responsibilities and stresses or a lack of motivation or due to your current circumstances. However, *feeling* sleepy is generally because you either didn't sleep so well the night before or that your body simply needs to sleep and recharge.

Both Margaret Thatcher and Donald Trump claimed to only require just four hours of sleep per night. We can't prove this, and if they did then I'd question how they were treating those around them whilst off camera? This I'll never know, but I do know that we all need more than that to restore and repair ourselves and function well.

According to the Guinness Book of Records, in 1997, they stopped monitoring the record for the longest time for anyone to stay awake. 'The record holder at the time was Robert McDonald, who went 453 hours 40 minutes (18 days 21 hours 40 minutes) without sleeping in 1986 (16). McDonald's record is not as well documented as Randy Gardner, who previously held the record in January 1964, when the17-year-old stayed awake for 11 days and 24 minutes.

The Guinness Book of Records said that 'we no longer monitor the record due to the inherent dangers associated with sleep deprivation, we can say that no one is known to have broken it since McDonald' (16). There you have it, the official record and the official reason why they are no longer accepting new records.

The Chernobyl disaster of 1986 and the Exxon Valdez oil spill of 1989 both occurred because the workers were sleep-deprived. These are well-documented, with the Chernobyl workers doing a 13-hour shift *without* a break. We are humans; *I-Robots* are thankfully not mainstream just yet. I am genuinely surprised that there are not more road accidents due to nightshift-workers returning home in the morning. Seriously, after a couple of 8-8 nightshifts with nearly an hour's drive home (thanks, rush-hour traffic) I'm just about nodding off about 5 miles from home, right when the traffic starts abruptly slowing down into Portsmouth. I chomp on chewing gum, fidget about in the seat, and wind both windows down - even when it is freezing in order to keep awake and to stay alive. I like to think that I'm a fairly responsible driver, and I don't play with my phone or have passenger distractions. How others (who I know do both) don't have accidents is beyond me. My reaction times, on occasion, must have been seriously reduced, and there are plenty of studies that concur. Sleep, as it so happens, is very underrated.

## HOW MUCH DO WE REALLY NEED?

It is well documented that adults need 7-9 hours per night, but we probably all knew that already. Shortly after my first child was born I was talking to my brother (who'd had three by then) as I was stressing about not getting enough sleep so he told me that you *can* survive on 6 hours' sleep. His dismissive attitude irritated me at first but this was actually quite reassuring; he was right, I could, and I did.

Getting 7-9 is far better, but stressing about not getting enough makes the golden ratio even more elusive. Let's face it, you survived when staying over and returning from a friend's house, when camping, holidays abroad, early hours trips to hospital etc. If you are so worried about the desynchrony of your delicate circadian rhythms that you only stray from the norm in an emergency then ask yourself if you are truly living. Worrying about disruption is usually far worse than the actual disruption itself.

Don't stress, you'll get there, make small adjustments, tweak your lifestyle and in time you'll either wonder why you had the problem, or begin to see the mistakes that were preventing you from getting a decent night's sleep.

# THE EPWORTH SLEEPINESS SCALE

*For my two teenage children, I would observe their weekend morning routines and label it 'The Hepworth Laziness Scale'. However, here is a well-documented assessment tool:*

The Epworth Sleepiness Scale is widely used in the field of sleep medicine as a subjective measure of a patient's sleepiness. The test is a list of eight situations in which you rate your tendency to become sleepy on a scale of 0, with no chance of dozing, to 3, high chance of dozing. When you finish the test, add up the values of your responses. Your total score is based on a scale of 0 to 24. The scale estimates whether you are experiencing excessive sleepiness that possibly requires medical attention.

**How Sleepy Are You?**

How likely are you to doze off or fall asleep in the following situations? You should rate your chances of dozing off, not just feeling tired. Even if you have not done some of these things recently try to determine how they would have affected you. For each situation, decide whether or not you would have:

**The Epworth Sleepiness Scale**

- No chance of dozing =0
- Slight chance of dozing =1
- Moderate chance of dozing =2
- High chance of dozing =3

Write down the number corresponding to your choice in the right-hand column. Total your score below.

| SITUATION | CHANCE OF DOZING |
|---|---|
| Sitting and reading | |
| Watching TV | |
| Sitting inactive in a public place (e.g., a theatre or a meeting) | |
| As a passenger in a car for an hour without a break | |
| Lying down to rest in the afternoon when circumstances permit | |
| Sitting and talking to someone | |
| Sitting quietly after a lunch without alcohol | |
| In a car, while stopped for a few minutes in traffic | |

Total Score = ______________________

**Analyse Your Score**

**Interpretation**

**0-7**: It is unlikely that you are abnormally sleepy.
**8-9:** You have an average amount of daytime sleepiness.
**10-15**: You may be excessively sleepy depending on the situation. You may want to consider
seeking medical attention.
**16-24**: You are excessively sleepy and should consider seeking medical attention.

*Reference: Johns MW. A new method for measuring daytime sleepiness: The Epworth Sleepiness Scale. Sleep 1991; 14(6):540-5.*

N.B. I have put a copy of the Epworth Sleepiness Scale at the back of this book to enable it to be photocopied if required.

# SLEEP APNOEA

Sleep apnoea is when your breathing stops and starts while you sleep, with the most common type being called obstructive sleep apnoea.

Some of the main symptoms include:

- Loud and chronic snoring.
- Choking or gasping during sleep.
- Witnessed pauses in breathing during sleep.
- Teeth grinding or clenching (bruxism).
- Frequent night-time awakenings and/or insomnia.

The following symptoms may all be experienced by someone with sleep apnoea, but may also be experienced by those who do not. They are a fair indication that one's sleep is not as it ought to be.

- Dry throat or mouth upon awakening. Either night or morning.
- Nocturnal palpitations, heartburn, racing heart rate or night sweats.
- Frequent urination during the night (nocturia).
- Noticeable daytime sleepiness.
- Morning headache.
- Short-term memory or learning problems.
- Poor concentration / attention / feeling irritable.
- Changes in mood, including feeling depressed.

**Common Causes**

- Being overweight and/or a large neck circumference.
- Abnormal upper airway anatomy (general ENT issues).
- Using medications, drugs, alcohol or smoking.
- Sleeping on the back, and/or REM sleep.

- Medical conditions such as heart failure, strokes, medications and various other long-term conditions, plus increased age.

Sleep apnoea is more common than people think, with approximately 22% of men and 17% of woman being affected. It is more common in men and is generally developed before the age of 65.

It is also worth noting that men measure their necks for clothing far more than women do, but what if the women reading this all rush out to measure their necks, what would the data show? That a thicker neck is likely to be indicative of the need to lose a few pounds, or that you're a wrestler like Butterbean? Seriously, we all know the generic healthcare advice of lose some weight and improve our fitness etc., so just start taking small steps to lead to a better you.

## CPAP = CONTINUOUS POSITIVE AIRWAY PRESSURE

When medical intervention is required, CPAP is the general treatment for obstructive sleep apnoea. The CPAP machine provides a constant flow of pressurized air that helps to maintain an open airway thus preventing collapse. The air is delivered via a fitted mask. It has been used to treat sleep apnoea since 1981. It is also effective in eliminating snoring, which usually occurs due to the vibration of the tissues in the throat (17).

**CPAP Machine**

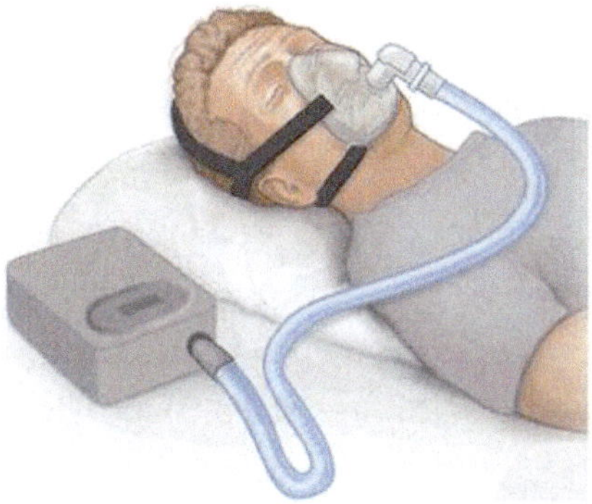

Basically, they take in room air, filter it, and blow it out via the mask. They are relatively quiet and either run on mains or rechargeable battery. Whoever provides the equipment will determine the setting that work best for you. There are also some masks that cover the nose only which some people prefer. Most models have an internal memory card to record data and can be analysed as required. Some CPAP machines also humidify the air.

## BIPAP= Bilevel Positive Airway Pressure

BiPAP basically offers a varying pressure during respirations, both inhaling and exhaling. This can be beneficial for those who have difficulty exhaling against the continuous pressure of CPAP. The machines and masks are pretty much the same.

## SLEEP TEST - POLYSOMNOGRAM

These are used to help diagnose sleep apnoea, restless leg syndrome (yes, there really is one) and other sleep disorders. These are performed at either a hospital sleep laboratory or at an outpatient sleep clinic. Your doctor should ask you and (if required) your partner about when and how you snore to help assess the severity of the problem. Some doctors ask their patients to write a 'self-report' that notes down the quality of sleep, how often they wake up, how rested they typically feel, and other issues. You may also have to have an X-ray, CT scan or MRI beforehand to assess the structure of your airways or ENT area.

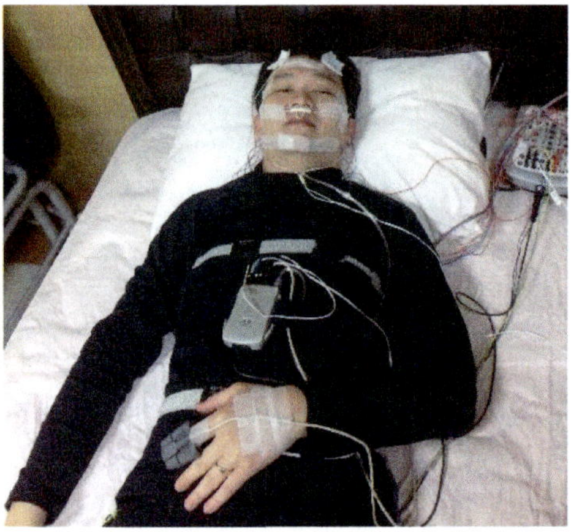

In a polysomnography, you're connected to many sensors and observed overnight. For the procedure, you'll have electrodes attached to the body to monitor brain waves, sleep stages and movement (including eyes and limbs). Other sensors will monitor the usual pulse, oxygen saturations and respirations, and your blood pressure and temperature are likely to be measured before and afterwards. Despite the drastic looking set-up (18), patients are not usually on oxygen or have tape on their chin. PJs, blankets and duvets are encouraged to allow for a more natural sleep.

Like everything medical, don't expect to get your results over your morning coffee. Sleep study reports are usually several pages long. It's not like an X-ray where you can see straightaway whether a bone is broken or not. Analysing the data takes time, and may need several professionals' input, so patience is key. Such a sleep test may be used to diagnose narcolepsy (excessive daytime sleepiness), which in itself can be confirmed by the 'Epworth Sleepiness Scale'. In simple terms, the sleep test will measure how well you slept, for how long, and how often you woke up. It also measures REM sleep and whether you are experiencing sleep apnoea, plus your pulse, respirations and oxygen levels in your blood.

## PARASOMNIA, OR ABNORMAL BEHAVIOUR DURING SLEEP

Although it's not always clear what causes parasomnias, they are thought to be linked to a condition; often emotional but sometimes physical, that will trigger strong feelings. This not only includes anxiety and fear but also things like happiness or sexual arousal.

General triggers include alcohol or drug use, overtiredness or exhaustion (possible accumulating insomnia / sleep-deprivation), anxiety, stress or depression, illness that can cause feverish sleep and also certain medications.

## SLEEP-TALKING

Talking in your sleep (the song of which was released in 1978 by Crystal Gayle), is medically known as somniloquy, and is a common sleep disorder characterized by unknowingly talking in your sleep. It is generally harmless, and can vary from senseless rambling to laughing and even shouting. More unnerving is that sleep-talkers can appear to be talking to themselves or engaging in a conversation with someone else as when they are awake. Thankfully, sleep-talkers have no recollection of their nocturnal talking episodes. This is usually only noticed once the individual shares a bed with someone, otherwise it can go unnoticed for years.

Sleep-talking can also be incidental, occurring only when a person is intoxicated or if they are sleep-deprived. For others, it can be a long-term condition during which they sleep-talk regularly, whether that's nightly or just several times a week. So, what do they actually talk about? Aforementioned, it's usually mindless babble that is merely a sentence or two, although it has been recorded as sometimes being threatening or explicit, with the use of profanities not necessarily associated with the person speaking.

Basically speaking, in stages 1-3 of sleep the sleep-talker may produce understandable conversation, which becomes more senseless or slurred as they move to a deeper sleep. By stage 4 of REM sleep when a person is actively dreaming they are not likely making sense to anyone overhearing them. However, sleep-talking isn't usually a problem until it interferes with the sleep of your partner.

If it is, then seek further help, and if you are going to see your GP then it's not a bad idea to show them a sleep journal. This doesn't have to be a War & Peace account of your entire life, just note down the timings of when you wake and sleep, how much you sleep, things that prevent your sleep, and your rough routine. You can use the chart at the back of this book as a guide. You don't need to stress about the timings either; getting up once in the night is fairly normal, but getting up every hour isn't. They don't need to know where you apply Ponds cold cream, but any alcohol and caffeine intake, exercise, sleep aids etc., would provide useful background information in assisting any diagnoses. If sleep-talking is bothering one of you, then earplugs, headphones or white noise machines may help.

## SLEEP-GROANING

Is medically known as catathrenia, and is, thankfully, rare. The sounds are often described as long moaning or humming whilst exhaling, which can also sound sexual in nature. Sleep-groaning can be in short sharp grunts or longer drawn-out moans and groans.

What is distressing for the bed-partner is the sheer unpredictability of the sounds, and that the groaner may appear either sad or sexually aroused, when neither is likely to be the case. Please remember that the person groaning is actually asleep, and will have no recollection of this when they wake up. Therefore, caution must be taken with recording such sounds on your phone and playing them back to your partner. You may unwittingly create a 'complex' with your partner which may lead to them developing insomnia, and thus both of you being in a worse scenario than before. Discuss it together first.

Sleep-groaning generally happens with younger people, hence the mistake that the sounds are sexual in nature. It could have been happening for years, and only noticed when sharing a bed with another person for the first time, or sleepovers, college, military digs etc. Thankfully it's not psychological or psychiatric in nature, even if it does sound a bit odd.

## SEXSOMNIA

Sexsomnia is basically sexual behaviour during sleep. They (never you, of course) could be fondling themself or their partner. It is more prevalent in men than in women and has led to clinical and relationship issues, and even legal consequences of such actions. With genuine sexsomnia, the person has no recollection of any events occurring as they were asleep. However, there is always potential for abuse, where people claim to have been asleep but were not, or are awake and actually had sex with their partner whilst their partner was asleep.

There are relational, moral, and legal ramifications for this subject, with many grey areas in between. What I would say is communicate with each other. It may not be as sinister as you may think, after all, your partner has no recollection upon waking. If the person who is making the advances is genuine then they will want to help to stop it, for the sake of the relationship. However, if in doubt, put barriers in place and get help, or if your safety is being compromised, then take whatever steps are necessary, from the spare room to even moving out.

## SLEEPWALKING

People often think that sleepwalking is funny, and the rise in popularity of YouTube and TikTok certainly glamorises and emphasises the amusing and random behaviour that is exhibited during sleepwalking episodes. However, this phenomenon has its risks and concerns, and having spoken to several people who have either sleepwalked or have known someone close who does, here is some advice to consider:

Firstly, bear in mind that their eyes are usually open whilst sleepwalking, although the person will look straight through people and not recognise them (because they are asleep!). They can often move well around familiar objects (19). However, it remains unclear whether the sleepwalker can actually see or not.

Try to steer the person back to bed, mainly for their safety, but also to prevent wall-to-wall carnage in your home. In the technological age that we now live in, please don't be so engrossed in capturing the moment on your phone that you overlook your chance to protect them. After all, whilst you are awake and they are not, you remain the responsible adult. One bad fall at the top of the stairs may make you TikTok famous for a minute but it could make your partner wheelchair bound for life.

Smaller children are easier to redirect, as they can usually be carried back to bed. For anyone else, it has been advised to steer their shoulders back to the direction of their bed and guide them there. For anyone showing signs of random behaviour (we know that all sleepwalking is unpredictable) then consider a bath towel looped around their arms as a type of restraint whilst guiding. This sounds a bit drastic but no-one wants a sucker-punch to the chops at 3am. Besides, you really are acting in their best interests by helping them return to bed.

I have personally met a man, in hospital, who had driven his car into a wall whilst sleep-driving. He did get a rude awakening, but thankfully his injuries were minor enough and that the police did not press any charges. No alcohol had been consumed. I thought that these stories were the subject of internet speculation, but this man had somehow collected his car keys, left his house, unlocked his car, put the keys in the ignition and then proceeded to randomly drive around, all whilst being asleep. He didn't get more than a few hundred metres from his house, but the fact that he got anywhere at all is both astonishing and worrying.

There have been several cases documented of sleep-driving with police involvement after a crash, such in the UK in 2011 where a GP lost his licence for a year due to sleep-driving as he crashed into some parked cars. Luckily for him he was in his PJs and dressing gown, as if he'd been in his regular clothes then it would have taken some believing. He was about four times over the drink-drive limit though, although it still seems a bit harsh that he had to admit drink driving when he had no recollection of this, AND was banned for a whole year. He informed the judge that from the incident onwards he locked all car keys away in a piano stool on the evenings when he had a drink (20).

So, do we need to be setting up cameras overnight to discover if we also sleepwalk? Not really, no. I assume that I do not sleepwalk, as this has never been observed throughout my childhood or marriage, but I have lived alone for a total of thirteen years, so it is possible, although everything has always been found as it was, so I think that it's highly unlikely. My mate Dan did, as a child, even going downstairs and wandering about, but this stopped when he reached his teenage years.

The following things can trigger sleepwalking or make it worse:

- Not getting enough sleep.
- Stress and anxiety.
- Infection with a high temperature, especially in children.
- Drinking too much alcohol or taking drugs.
- Certain types of medicine, such as some sedatives.
- Being startled by a sudden noise or touch, causing abrupt waking from deep sleep.
- Waking up suddenly from deep sleep because you need to go to the toilet.
- Restless leg syndrome (21).

# SLEEP PARALYSIS

Sleep paralysis is when you cannot move or speak as you are waking up or falling asleep. It can be scary but it's harmless and most people will only get it once or twice in their life (22). Between 8% and 50% of people experience sleep paralysis at some point during their life. About 5% of people have regular episodes. Males and females are affected equally. Sleep paralysis has been described throughout history (22).

It is believed to have played a role in the creation of stories about alien abduction and other paranormal events. Many people from differing religious or spiritual backgrounds believe that it is either demonic or has some form of spiritual connotation to it. If you type 'sleep paralysis' into Google images then there are drawings of people with belts wrapped around their torso or 'monsters' crouching on top of people's chests.

The research suggests that individuals seem to have these same characteristics:

- Being awake but unable to move, speak, or open their eyes.
- The feeling that someone is in their room.
- The feeling that something is pushing them down.
- Feeling terrified (23).

Whoever experiences it complains of excessive fear which does not appear limited to the fact that the individual cannot move at all. The feelings can last for several minutes, but the sensation generally feels far longer due to the disturbing feeling of being totally out of control. This can also creep someone out for quite a while once awake and able to move about. There is no clear-cut documentation as to the cause of it either, which is a bit disconcerting. The jury's out on its cause and effect. I have my theories but so do the X-Files, so I'll leave this one here. I pray that you don't ever experience it.

# NARCOLEPSY

Narcolepsy is where the brain is unable to regulate sleeping and waking patterns normally, therefore the person cannot always choose when to be awake or asleep. People with narcolepsy may fall asleep without warning. Obviously this could be very dangerous and thankfully this condition is rare. It is thought to be a long-term condition, although people have been known to adjust their lifestyles to significantly reduce the symptoms, but it still poses some dangers. Some people may become socially isolated or withdrawn to avoid embarrassing themselves or impacting others. Possible triggers of narcolepsy include: hormonal changes or major psychological stress. It is thought to affect men and women equally.

Narcolepsy may be caused by a lack of the brain chemical hypocretin (AKA orexin), which regulates wakefulness. The lack of hypocretin is thought to be caused by autoimmunity, and attacking the cells that produce it or the receptors that allow it to work. However, this does not explain all cases of narcolepsy, and the exact cause of the problem is uncertain.

The common symptoms are:

- Excessive daytime sleepiness – feeling very drowsy throughout the day and finding it difficult to concentrate and stay awake.
- Sleep attacks – falling asleep suddenly and without warning.
- Cataplexy – temporary loss of muscle control resulting in weakness and possible collapse, often in response to emotions such as laughter and anger.
- Sleep paralysis, which a temporary inability to move or speak when waking up or falling asleep.

- Excessive dreaming and waking in the night – dreams often come as you fall asleep (hypnogogic hallucinations) or just before or during waking (hypnopompic hallucinations) (24).

It is estimated to affect about 30,000 people in the UK (the UK population being 68.9m in May 2023).

## SOME SCIENCEY BITS

Gamma-aminobutyric acid (GABA) is an amino acid that serves as the primary inhibitory neurotransmitter in the brain and a major inhibitory neurotransmitter in the spinal cord (25). GABA is the main neurotransmitter of the Central Nervous System (CNS), and it is well established that activation of GABA receptors promotes sleep. Sleep-promoting neurons in the anterior hypothalamus release GABA. This inhibits wake-promoting regions in the hypothalamus and in the brainstem. Adenosine also promotes sleep by inhibiting wakefulness-promoting neurons localized to the basal forebrain, lateral hypothalamus, and tuberomammillary nucleus (26).

The transitions between sleep and waking states are orchestrated by multiple brain structures, which include:

**Hypothalamus:** this controls the onset of sleep, and helps to regulate the circadian rhythm.

**Hippocampus**: is the memory region that is active during dreaming.

**Amygdala**: is the emotion centre that is active during dreaming.

**Thalamus**: this prevents the sensory signals from reaching the cortex.

**Reticular formation:** regulates the transition between your sleep and wakefulness (26).

**Amygdala:** The amygdala is the centre for emotions, emotional behaviour, decision-making, social behaviour, motivation and memory formation. I have included it here because a malfunctioning or damaged amygdala can cause emotional and behavioural symptoms, such as increased irritability, strong emotions and confusion. With the amygdala being responsible for the perception of emotions such as anger, fear and sadness, so changes or imbalances may well lead to aggression or aggressive behaviour. It also helps to store memories of emotions and events to enable future recognition.

The bad news is that caffeine stimulates the amygdala, not unlike cortisol, therefore amplifying the fight or flight response and intensifying any sense of threat (27). Anxiety is the obvious symptom, but depression is also directly linked; possibly because the individual is anxious but does not necessarily know why. See the section on caffeine for more details.

**Adenosine**: Is produced naturally in the body and is a neurotransmitter, and our neutrons (nerve cells) are imbedded with adenosine receptors. Adenosine is often found with a molecule called adenosine triphosphate (ATP). ATP is considered the 'energy currency' of cells, as it stores and provides energy. When adenosine binds to these receptors, a variety of proteins that inhibit neurons are released. This suppression of nerve cell activity is what causes the feeling of *drowsiness.* As a person expends energy and the ATP is metabolised throughout the day, adenosine is released as a byproduct. The longer you stay awake, the more adenosine accumulates and the sleepier you gradually become. (26). Adenosine is an inhibitory neurotransmitter, meaning that it acts as a central nervous system depressant and inhibits many processes associated with wakefulness. It has a similar affect to alcohol on the body.

**Pons:** The pons is located where your brain joins with your spinal cord, and is part of your brainstem. One of its jobs is to handle the 'unconscious processes' such as breathing and your sleep-wake cycle, and helps to initiate REM sleep. It is possibly where we get the term *ponder* from?

## THE SUMMARY

There is a lot of research about what part of the brain does what and the relevant professors and scholars will no doubt inform you in great detail, with this part of the brain doing this, and why this part interacts with that part etc. Personally, I'm not entirely convinced that the neurophysicists and professors truly know how we sleep because I don't think that it was designed to be discovered. It's not like digestion where food goes in and waste comes out. It just is what it is.

There are so many variables to getting a good night's sleep, and there are many neurochemicals that are secreted and processed by the brain. The brain also processes so much throughout the day, and any slight chemical imbalance for a whole variety of different situations and reasons could cause some form of sleep impairment.

## THE TANGENT

There are also childhood traumas that can trigger anxiety unknowingly, causing sporadic sleep loss, making pattern-forming hard, therefore more complex in tackling the variables as they are unpredictable. Many people associate childhood traumas with some form of physical abuse. However, abuse is not just physical. Experiences such as being shouted at, humiliated, bullied, neglected or rejected can all cause deep inner wounds that manifest randomly causing anxiety that can be totally unrelated to the experiences of the day. Try writing down how you view yourself emotionally, physically, sexually, spiritually, relationally, socially and reflect on your findings (physically is the easiest as long as you are realistic; I'll never compete for strongmen competitions as I'm not big enough). Be realistic, but be kind to yourself, then take whatever small steps you can to improve.

Work out the negative aspects and ask a friend/relative/partner for help and advice to see how you can improve them. They probably view you in a far better way than you view yourself. The negative viewpoints from your self-analysis are probably areas that need some work, whether it be family/friends who could support you or by getting professional help. Write down positive affirmations, deal with your past and the anxiety will subside. Even if you're not an anxious person, look at your list and improve if you're not happy with it. Your sleep will get better if you deal with your inner mud.

# CHAPTER 5
# CHEMICAL COSH

*"I'm for anything that gets you through the night, be it prayer, tranquilisers, or a bottle of Jack Daniels"* - Frank Sinatra.

## ALCOHOL

*Use everything in moderation, including moderation!* - Oscar Wilde

Anyone who has consumed alcohol will appreciate (or not) its effects on the body. Many people think that it is a stimulant, but it's really a central nervous system depressant, eventually causing the body to slow down and stop. Drinking slows down the way that your senses process information therefore *lowering your inhibitions* by default. So, alcohol reduces inhibitions thereby giving confidence at the same time. A dangerous combination. Hence why half-respectable people can be seen dancing on the tables before midnight. What seemed like a great idea at the time may not be quite so good the following day. At the police station, or even worse; but don't tell.

It is easy to think that you'll have a great night's sleep by having plenty to drink. You just hit the sack and lights out until morning. That's if you're lucky and even then, your sleep won't have been as fulfilling as if you'd left the booze alone. For the unlucky ones, you may crash out immediately, but wake up just a few hours later, take the inevitable toilet break, chug some water and a couple of paracetamol and settle into bed for a restless night. Many people overheat and get the night sweats as your liver is working at full capacity processing all that alcohol (worse still with a doner kebab inside you as well) and you're burning up. If you need a bucket by your bedside then perhaps you need to evaluate your lifestyle choices, but I bet most people have had a bucket there at some point in their lives.

The alcohol in your system will mean you spend less time in the important Rapid Eye Movement (REM) stage of sleep (the restorative phase) meaning that you wake up feeling less refreshed (28). It makes sense that you have more slow-wave or deep sleep due to the sedative factor of the alcohol, but that doesn't make for a well-rested night.

Drinking every day is not good for anyone, whatever some people may say. Consider making your last drink 2-3 hours before bed, this may work for you, and would certainly improve your sleep, if you can. I see hangovers as my body's way of having a dirty protest that I've poisoned it the night before and it's reminding me not to do it again any time soon, and my body seems to focus its attention to my head for maximum impact.

Some of the best night's sleep that I had was in 2022 in my mid-forties when I stopped all alcohol and caffeine (apart from tea) for two months in the summer and was training hard. However, I've also downed a large Scotch or vodka late evening when I've been stressed or overwhelmed and my mind has been on overdrive, with great results; particularly after a 12-hour shift. It takes the edge off my edginess and settles me down *quickly*. So, should you avoid alcohol altogether? To get a better night's sleep, probably. As a reward? You deserve a treat. Socially; definitely not. However, I did sleep a lot better without it after a few days.

## NICOTINE AND CANNABIS

Nicotine IS a stimulant, as it causes the body to release adrenaline (epinephrine) and yet is also an anxiolytic, reducing anxiety and anger, therefore providing a sedative effect by default. What a paradox! Nicotine is found in the nightshade family of plants, including peppers, tomatoes, potatoes and aubergines (eggplants) and is a naturally produced alkaloid, most highly concentrated in the tobacco plant. You can make a pesticide out of nicotine, and it can also be used to poison someone.

For those who use tobacco products in the evening, the nicotine hit is not going to help you get to sleep. It is also noted that smokers are statistically likely to drink more caffeine (29). However, to make lasting changes in life, go one step at a time, and if you've always had a smoke just before bed then try some of the other tips in this book first, then as you start to feel better you can consider adjusting your smoking times. When you're in a better place you could make your last cigarette half an hour before bed, then an hour and progress that way over time. This should start to improve your quality of sleep. I could just say, 'just stop today' but that's not helpful to you at the moment, so make a plan to reduce the time of your last smoke progressively. Some people do just go cold turkey, but this is rare, and in order to make lasting changes it is better to start small.

Cannabis can help you sleep, but is it a healthy option? It could be argued, by some, that gaining the overall nourishment of sleep outweighs the negative effects of cannabis use (lung damage, potential psychosis). I sit on the fence on this one. There are legal implications of growing your own and/or distributing it here in the UK, so I'm not likely to advocate it for growing, using or selling. Just be aware that if you're stoned off your toots and sitting up in bed trying not to puke then that's not helpful. The main point is that if you already enjoy using cannabis and then you are not likely to listen to what anyone else says anyway, because it's what you do, so if it works then great, I'm happy for you.

There is, however, good news on the smoking front, as there are several kinds of plants that can be smoked that do not contain any nicotine and have negligible tar content. Herbs such as mullein, damiana, marshmallow leaf, dried mint and chamomile can all be smoked. I'll let you go down that rabbit hole of smokable herbs, most available on eBay, and only about a fiver for 100g! Perfect for a night out when you crave a smoke but don't want a nicotine hit/craving, or as a base for a bifta, or just want to sit and have a ponder by a fire every now and then with a pipe. As with all smoking, there is a risk of lung cancer and COPD, and I've seen many cases of both first-hand, and it's not pretty. None of the patients thought that it would happen to them, and I've often said to my mate that if his next cigarette would cause a tumour like on the tobacco packet pictures then would he still smoke it? I think we all know the answer to that, but we did it anyway. Not good, however infrequently we indulge, so I'll leave it on your moral compass, but at least there are 'healthier' tobacco alternatives available as above.

In the UK there are many CBD or hemp shops that have a wide range of oils available that can help you to relax without getting high.

## SLEEPING TABLETS

Zopiclone, Zolpidem and Clomethiazole, are Prescription Only Medications (POM) in the UK, with Zopiclone being the most common. In darker days past I went to my GP and got a prescription for Zopiclone as I was struggling with everything, which was causing insomnia by default, but thankfully this was over a decade ago. 3.75mg was enough to get me off to sleep, but if you're particularly 'muscular' or neurotic then the 7.5mg dose may be more beneficial. Always ask for the 7.5mg anyway, because you can half the tablet so you'll get twice as many for the cost of your prescription. You're welcome.

Please bear in mind that ALL sleeping tablets, whether POM or Over The Counter (OTC) medications whilst not technically addictive are likely to create dependence, which is a bit like addiction by default. Despite some people being on them for ever, they are best kept as a short-term plan. As a guideline, I'd suggest a few weeks/months to get over a 'bad patch' and then form a plan to wean yourself off them. Unless you like being dependent on 'the system' or being dependent on pills; if so then aim to stay on them for ever.

## MORPHINE

Morphine-based painkillers are a Prescription Only Medication (POM) in the UK and generally have the side-effect of drowsiness and respiratory depression. The main opioid/morphine-based medications are: MST, Zomorph, Sevredol, Morphgesic, Oramorph, hydrocodone, oxycodone, oxymorphone, plus codeine-based analgesia.

## BENZODIAZEPINES

These are a Prescription Only Medication (POM) in the UK, so only available via a hospital or your GP practice. They are sedative medications and therefore create a sense of dependence and even addiction, and may require a withdrawal programme once no longer required. Temazepam Diazepam, Lorazepam, Clobazam, Clonazepam, Nitrazepam are some of the more common BZDPs available in the UK.

## MELATONIN

Is also a Prescription Only Medication (POM) in the UK. However, as it is legal in many countries as an OTC medication and it can be obtained online. Caution should be taken if using vitamin D supplements, as they may suppress melatonin production hence why melatonin is a POM, to stop people self-medicating without taking a holistic approach, and without knowing the contraindications. So, what exactly is melatonin? It is a hormone that is produced by the brain in response to darkness, and helps with the timing of your internal body-clock (circadian rhythms) and therefore sleep. Melatonin production can be blocked by being exposed to light at night.

# OVER THE COUNTER (OTC) MEDICATIONS

All OTC medications that cause drowsiness must be kept behind the counter in the UK, and cannot be bought without a brief discussion with a staff member. In my experience, these staff members fall into three categories:

1) They are ex-military/know-it-all/narcissistic psychopaths who will take pleasure in interrogating you and giving their own form of advice, and will often withhold the item that you've requested in order to retain power over you.
2) This type doesn't care at all. They are indifferent to your presence, and would happily sell you 100 paracetamol if they could.
3) They care. They smile at you and respect your intelligence and understanding of the product that you are buying. They may ask minimal questions, but only because they have to. They are warm to be around and we need more of them in this world.

**Night Nurse** Contains an antihistamine called promethazine which is generally used as a sedative. Pharmacy staff are more reluctant to sell this to people who just want to get to sleep as it contains other medications that if not required are not beneficial to take; as dictated to by our shop assistant in category 1). I have used Night Nurse before with good effect for short-term colds/insomnia mix.

**Phenergan** Also contains promethazine which is a better choice if sleep is your only issue.

**Nytol** Contains diphenhydramine which is an antihistamine (allergy relief). It is generally more sedating than other antihistamines.

**Piriton** Contains chlorphenamine, which is also an antihistamine. It is well known for its sedating properties; therefore caution is required with it for daily use. Generally, not sold to assist with sleeping, but for some, its use has been beneficial.

The non-drowsy tablets are considered relaxing rather than sedating, and are available from most supermarkets and chemists and are available without interrogation.

**Kalm's, Sominex** and a herbal type of **Nytol**. Their main ingredients are a mixture of valerian, hops and passion flower. Then there's Rescue Remedy, which is an anti-anxiety potion available as a spray, drops or pastilles. It is made up of flowers that I can't pronounce or spell, but it gets rave reviews. Amazon customers are known to be quite savage if things don't work, but out of 13,000+ reviews, 73% give Rescue Remedy 5 stars AND a decent write up, with only 3% giving a 1 star, so there's definitely something in it that works. I believe that one of the plants is called Placebous Soporifica, harvested on the eastern side of the land of Nod.

**Melatonin in milk** I'd love to say that this was just for fun, but there really is milk that has been collected from cows that have been milked pre-dawn. The theory is that there is more melatonin in the milk and will therefore assist you getting to sleep after consuming it. However, the online forum called 'Mumsnet' suggests that after randomized controlled trials there was no real conclusive benefit to such a milk. Lullaby Milk in Ireland would disagree, and have the science to back it up, so they could be worth checking out.

There are so many herbal supplements that are available in various forms, such as powders, pills or as teabags. As an Englishman, I find that an evening tisane can be most agreeable, and most forms of herbal tea are beneficial, but avoid ginseng ones in the evening. Go for a 'sleepy' tea bag and tell yourself that they are helping you to sleep and they will. Generally.

**L-theanine** is found primarily in green and black tea and some mushrooms, and is an amino acid. Available to purchase as pills, it promotes relaxation by reducing stress and anxiety levels. Available online and via health food stores.

**Ashwagandha** is worth considering and there is a ton of research out there on it. It is supposed to calm you down and make you less neurotic. There's a man who goes by the name of Pigmie who has a great YouTube channel, and he tried it for 30 days and charted his discoveries (https://www.youtube.com/watch?v=IX4IDfW-SuEY&t=94s *or simply type in: Pigmie Ashwagandha 30 days*). Granted people may respond differently but his results were very interesting. It is also a testosterone booster (possibly by default, as it reduces prolactin production in the pituitary). There's a deep rabbit hole of research and findings, but if interested then his video is worth checking out.

**Hops** needs little introduction as it is an ingredient in all beers (apart from gruit). Even alcohol-free beer that has a high hops content has been known to make people sleepy. Again, lots of available research out there; it can be purchased online and via health food stores in the form of powders, pills and teabags. Works for many, but not for all, so try some and see how you go.

**Magnesium** is supposed to promote sleep by relaxing muscles therefore reducing stress and promoting calmness. Try Epsom salts in a bath to increase magnesium levels. For supplements, there is a wide variety of doses available and recommended. Body sprays are better than tablets due to the faster absorption rate. When I started using it years ago it used to itch like crazy; a sure sign that my magnesium levels were low. With persistence, the levels increased and the itching stopped. I put it down to my pink salt intake but the jury's out on this. Magnesium-rich foods include green leafy vegetables, nuts and seeds, although soil depletion can reduce the mineral content. Suffice to say that magnesium has numerous roles within the body and low levels mean a less well functioning body.

**Smint & Tic-Tacs** Are sweets, not sleeping tablets. However, the brain is a powerful force, and you may be able to persuade yourself that by taking a nightly Smint with a sip of water may be just the thing to settle your mind and trick yourself into falling asleep. I've taken paracetamol for a headache/cold and I've 'placeboed' myself into believing that I will sleep very well because of them. Of course I know that this is not the case with paracetamol, but there is something very powerful about this activity, as I 'trick' my brain into settling and sleeping. Give the Smints a try. They might just work and at least you've got something on hand for the morning breath.

So, whether you need to see a GP for some sleeping tablets, or fancy trying some OTC antihistamines, or simply having a happy herbal brew then go for it. Whether you use ashwagandha or ashfromganja, experiment to find what works for you.

## DISCLAIMER 1:

*It is not advisable to combine alcohol with any form of sleeping tablet mentioned in this section as it could increase the sedative effect. Just because I have had good results taking Piriton (or other OTC tablets at different times) with a large Scotch does not mean that I would advise or condone it. The alcohol and medications may work in synergy to create a drowsier state, which could be dangerous, so once again, I do not advise doing so.*

# DISCLAIMER 2:

*Many of the BZDP's, codeine and Zopiclone can be obtained via online pharmaceuticals and some steroid websites. They can also be bought easily from chemists abroad, often within, or just outside the EU. I do not condone such practices, nor could I advise your work colleagues to collect some for you the next time they go abroad. Neither would I advise you to 'try one out' to see if they work for you, from a friend or relative. These can be dangerous medications and I must therefore advise you to be a responsible citizen and contact your GP for all medical advice.*

# CHAPTER 6
# MENTAL HEALTH

*If there is no enemy within, the enemy outside can do you no harm* African Proverb.

Apparently, more women than men are diagnosed with anxiety disorders and depression. It could be argued that it's because women are reaching out more and getting the help that they need. It is statistically proven that more men commit suicide than women which could be because men simply aren't reaching out enough. Some possible reasons why men don't ask for help is because people may laugh at them or perceive them as being weak. Men's egos are fragile and experiences like ridicule and rejection can be quite damaging to some (and if you kick against this statement then you are not as secure in your masculinity as you need to be). Other reasons include not wanting to bother other people, being too busy or being oblivious to the fact that you may actually need help.

Current affairs in the UK are not great at present. The cost-of-living crisis, with food, fuel and heating all causing financial problems to many UK households, alongside the backdrop of a certain world-wide event that started in 2020 (so I'm only going to repeat the expected narrative here) has got many people into a state of somewhat fevered anxiety. Enter the Central Bank Digital Currency (CBDC) and soon the Unicoin (a strange mythical coin of universal value that may replace all global currencies; research it) plus an impending microchip in our hands that has all our medical records on (for our safety, of course) and that we can also make all our CBDC payments with (which is happening in parts of Sweden already). Remember that it is all part of a global plan to reduce carbon dioxide (unless you're already in the club). Rather than swapping beef for bugs, I do my bit by refusing to have my own private jet.

Recent technological advances have managed to make wind-turbine powered ships though. Wind-powered ships? Who'd have thought? What a time to be alive! Sail away… Our future sounds unique as we pioneer into the 4th Industrial Revolution, but have no fear, because according to the WEF, 'by 2030, we will own nothing and be happy'. Thankfully for me I'm already there. However, this impending dystopian utopia and the aftermath of the uniqueness of Covid-19 has left a few people struggling to sleep. Not surprising considering the current concerns like a lack of Russian vodka (thanks to woke supermarket boycotts), and whether robots will take over our jobs.

Cogitating, reflecting, ruminating, contemplating, mulling, deliberating, chewing the cud (linked to ruminating, as the cud is stored in the rumen chamber of the animal's stomach, in case you wondered), everyone needs a good old ponder every now and then. However, if you are worried about the future and reflecting on the past then you'll miss out on each day-to-day moment. Living in the present is a phenomenon now known as mindfulness.

# EMOTIONS

Happiness can be pursued, it's rarely found if strived after and it is usually best when it happens naturally, but how do we get more of it? One man's coffee is another man's tea, so let's look at a few opposites of happiness:

*Depression, despair, discouragement, displeasure, dissatisfaction, gloom, melancholy, misery, sadness, discontent, sorrow.*

Not a pretty picture, I know. That said, if you work at these areas in your life and find out what the triggers are that make you feel unhappy and write them down then you'll have something to work with and work through, either privately, with a close friend or with professional help. In my profession I'm probably supposed to say 'get professional help', but just telling a mate is a step in the right direction. We don't all need psychotherapy, so find what works for you and reach out. People who bottle it all up are rarely the epitome of happiness and fulfilment. Deal with your inner junk and happiness will come by default. Don't strive at it, enjoy the process, but don't spend too much time in the past, as your future is yet to be enjoyed.

When going through a difficult time I feel afraid to ask for a hug, or some money for short-term help, or some advice on a decision, or that I need a break from some of the chaos at work. Having someone to listen to us to get something off our chests is very underrated. Some men tragically take their own lives due to the perception and reality that women want a 'strong man'. It's hard to be perceived as weak or for needing help, so many of us keep going, constantly striving to get ourselves out of whatever mess we may find ourselves in. However, some people are simply in denial of their own shortcomings until it's too late. As above: *Deal with your inner junk, reach out and get help, and happiness will come by default.*

The Dalai Lama, when asked what surprised him most about humanity, answered:

*"Man, because he sacrifices his health in order to make money. Then he sacrifices money to recuperate his health. And then he is so anxious about the future that he does not enjoy the present; the result being that he does not live in the present or the future; he lives as if he is never going to die, and then dies having never really lived."*

Jesus Christ said, *"Therefore, do not worry about tomorrow, for tomorrow will worry about its own things. Sufficient for the day is its own trouble."*

Brilliant wisdom right here, but really, it's just common sense, so try to be present in each moment, or at least at some point within your day. Develop an 'attitude of gratitude'. Seriously, there are many people who will go to bed hungry tonight, and many who do not have the luxury nor safety that you are experiencing right now. We all know that the 'celebrities' probably sleep in a better bed and in a nicer room than we do, but that's THEIR life, not yours. Enjoy what you have, be grateful and enjoy the feelings of appreciation in what you have; being appreciative leads to simple contentment. Happiness will come as you reach out to help others too; often when and where you'd least expect it.

## WAKING UP, OR JUST CAN'T SLEEP

Stress is counter-productive to most things, and not surprisingly, to sleep too. If you've already tried everything that you can think of, and the military method had left you more tensed and ready for a battle than being relaxed, then put simply: don't stress about it. Easier said than done, I know. Enjoy your time lying in bed and resting. Reflect on your day, use a notepad if required to de-clutter your mind. Make some basic plans such as what to eat the next day, or something equally trivial that requires little thought yet keeps the brain occupied. That way you'll tire your brain out and be productive at the same time.

Even if you don't fall asleep immediately you will still get the benefit of resting. Granted it is not as restorative as actual sleep, but it really is better than nothing, and better than doomscrolling the night away, so make it your goal to enjoy it. You will probably need to re-train your mind to look at the lack of sleep in a positive way (of course it isn't a positive thing, but looking at it as a negative is a much worse option). The fear of being awake causes enough anxiety to stress you into the fight or flight mode, producing the usual cocktail of stress hormones. These can take some time to subside, and then being worried that late is the hour can bring them all back again. Insomnia can be a vicious circle.

*"Paradoxical intention can also be applied in cases of sleep disturbance. The fear of sleeplessness results in a hyper-intention to fall asleep, which, in turn, incapacitates the patient to do so. To overcome this particular fear, I usually advise the patient not to try to sleep but rather to try to do just the opposite, that is, to stay awake as long as possible. In other words, the hyper-intention to fall asleep, arising from the anticipatory anxiety of not being able to do so, must be replaced by the paradoxical intention not to fall asleep, which soon will be followed by sleep."*
*— Viktor E. Frankl, Man's Search for Meaning*

So do something simple that makes you happy! As soon as you switch your mindset and be happy with the fact that you are resting and doing some 'gentle thinking and planning' then that action in itself will reduce your cortisol and allow you to be in a much better place to fall asleep. It is also Sod's law that when you want to lie there resting and planning your next day or the weekend that you'll probably fall asleep anyway, so you've achieved your sleep by default.

For those early hours after an all-too-brief sleep, it is wise to plan a solution rather than lying awake questioning why you can't sleep. Have headphones and an MP3 player available. I'd avoid your phone as the temptation to jump on the social media platforms will be great, and then the doomscrolling truly begins. Have a book available, although an enthralling novel may not be the best option. Cookery, gardening or random travel books are entertaining enough but are not generally too gripping. Personally, I stay away from such erotica as Rosemary Conley's 'Hip and Thigh Diet' as I find it far too racy. You could also give the old insomnia a poke in the eye by using any awake time to recite some positive affirmations to yourself. This way you use the time wisely to build yourself up, despite the temporary setback of being awake. Marcus Aurelius is a fair place to start, as is YouTube, the internet etc. Alternatively, just for fun, you could take everything that you loathe and despise about yourself and speak the absolute opposite straight to your heart. You may be surprised at how negatively you view yourself, and how positive that you can become in just one night. With this knowledge, maybe your next early morning insomnia will happen for a reason? Spend your time wisely, and become the best person that you can be.

Consider watching a comedy film/episode before bed, as laughter releases all sorts of 'feel good' chemicals such as dopamine, serotonin and endorphins. Go for slapstick type comedy such as Charlie Chaplin or Jeeves & Wooster where you can just laugh at the simplicity of the moment rather than the highly intellectual type of comedy that may set your mind into overdrive

If this doesn't appeal, then give your biggest and silliest smile. Try it now; crack a smile as you read this, hold it for a few seconds and you'll start to feel better. Weird, isn't it? Even a fake smile will work to elevate your mood, even when you don't feel like it. The challenge is to try it at 3am when you've woken up and start to feel snotty about everything. If you can remember to, then keep smiling.

## STAYING IN BED WHEN YOU CAN'T SLEEP?

This is a contentious issue as most sleep books, journals etc., will advise getting up, then returning to bed when you get sleepy again. The theory there is that by lying in bed awake and restless your mind can associate being in bed as being in a negative place where you simply toss and turn for hours. Therefore, remove yourself from there, eat, drink and be merry and then return once you're sleepy again. However, the experts haven't taken into account the fuel crisis and that many people's homes in winter are freezing cold overnight.

However, if I wake up at 3am and my mind is racing then I find it better to get up and potter about or even go for a walk, because if I'm lying in bed tossing and turning then I'll get stressy which is likely to make me short-fused all day. Stressy and snotty: a winning combination for a rough day.

I generally take a happy compromise and go and make a herbal tea, maybe have a light bite to eat, grab a book, hunker down under the duvet and read until my eyes get heavy again. That way I'm in prime position to switch off the light and salvage what hours that I have left.

## BRITISH SUMMER TIME: THE DREADED CLOCK-SWITCH

Twice a year in the UK parents of young children dread the adjusting of the clocks, whether to Spring-Forward or Fall-Back an hour, as that one-hour difference plays havoc with our daily routines. Teenagers are not immune either, notably in the springtime, with their defiant protests at 10pm of 'it's really only 9pm though.' Try waking them an hour earlier the next day and their defiance will quickly ebb. Every action has an equal and opposite reaction…

The clocks change in March to make the most of increased summer daylight hours in the northern hemisphere. I think most people would be happy to make March the last ever clock change and leave it at that, but alas, it continues. The hour of disruption is well documented, and can affect farming, the stock market and air transport, although we've all just learnt to deal with it. RoSPA (Royal Society for the Prevention of Accidents) has campaigned against the clock change for years, the main priority being for cyclists' and pedestrians' road safety. Apparently 59 percent of British people would prefer BST all year round, according to a YouGov survey in 2019 (30).

To minimise the disruption, and to cut through all the fluff, go for the middle time, by simply adding or subtracting half an hour either off or onto your bedtime. Job done. Your children will say you're being mean, and technically you are, but do this each clock change and you'll all reset to the hour difference within a few sleeps. Simplicity is key. You can do this in shorter 15-minute increments if required, but most people, including children, can adapt easily to a half an hour change. You may be disrupted for a day or two, but alas, this is a part of life.

## CALMING THE MIND

Stress is well-documented as being one of the main reasons why people can't sleep. The stress is usually due to having a busy mind. When you try to block the thoughts out they seem to come back thick and fast, or be replaced by other thoughts. Not good. so how do we block them out? In short, you don't, write them down instead. Sometimes I have been unable to get to sleep and had to write things down in order to remain sane, and on reflection, it could have all been avoided. How? By prioritising a 'brainstorm' with pen and paper earlier in the evening. Granted, we all have appointments, clubs etc., but if I had have not watched that film or YouTube or whatever I was doing and sat down at 8pm for an hour and had a brainstorm then my mind would have been much clearer by bedtime. Most of it comes down to my 'me time' and priorities. Many people demand this as their 'right' and then wonder why they can't sleep later on.

Life goes in cycles and we all have different seasons. During my stressful or busy times, I HAD to journal/brainstorm, otherwise I'd probably have had a nervous breakdown. You may sometimes have to miss out on social events etc., but if your sanity and survival are at stake then it's a small price to pay, and Fear Of Missing Out (FOMO) is only temporary anyway.

## CHANGE YOUR MINDSET

Nearly every self-made millionaire has changed theirs. Believe that you will sleep and you will. I sometimes say out loud that I will sleep well tonight. Frame your world with your voice. There is life and death in the power of the tongue. You have the power to achieve this by your belief and by your spoken word. See the Sleep Affirmations section in Chapter 10.

# CHAPTER 7
# CAFFEINE

Caffeine is the most widely used psychoactive compound, is an adenosine receptor antagonist, which simply means that it blocks adenosine receptors in the brain, blocking drowsiness and therefore promoting wakefulness by default. Caffeine also enhances the release of acetylcholine, which is a neurotransmitter that communicates signals between the neurons and the central nervous system (CNS).

## So, what does this mean for me?

If you are prone to a poor night's sleep for whatever reasons, then allow plenty of time between your last cup of coffee and lights out. This is subjective, and trial and error will dictate what works for you. My sleep is quite good now, but I still consume my last 'leaded' coffee before 2pm, with a bedtime of 10pm therefore leaving 8 hours to leave my system. When a good night's sleep was more of a challenge, I only had one cup with a 10am cut-off. That said, you have to find what works for you, and avoiding caffeine altogether for a certain time may work for the best. If you're desperate to sleep then you'll do it.

The average cup of coffee contains about 80-100mg caffeine. It lasts for four to six hours on average, but has a half-life of another three to seven hours, depending on the individual. Therefore, a large coffee can have up to 200mg caffeine, which means that you will have up to 100mg still in your system about five hours later. Yikes! That means that you'll potentially have 50mg cruising through your system ten hours later, and that's based on only one cup a day! It can take up to twelve hours for caffeine to fully leave your system.

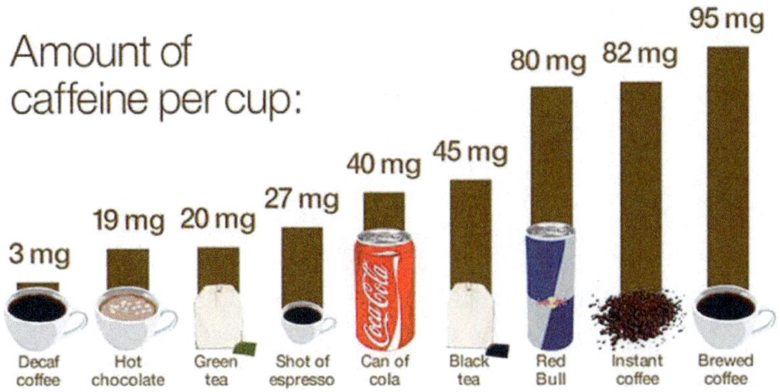


Image: *https://www.billi-uk.com/news/caffeine-content-favourite-drinks/*

Having researched both Monster and Red Bull, each 500ml can contains about 160mg of caffeine. Caffeine is also found in chocolate.

Like everything else, human beings are complex and we all produce varying levels of adenosine, and therefore metabolise caffeine at slightly different rates.

Also, the timing of our last caffeine intake will vary, so the effects will differ from one person to another, hence why some people can have a cup of coffee just before bed and still sleep well. However, the mind is very powerful, and worrying about your caffeine intake timing could lead to a much worse night's sleep than consuming the actual caffeine itself.

**Quick funny story:** Whilst working in a hospital, I went to a dear lady's (in her eighties) bedside at the start of my morning shift to ask her how she was, and she replied that she felt terrible and that she hadn't slept all night. I noticed an empty can of Red Bull on her bedside table and asked her what time she drank it. 'Well, right before bed' was the answer that the poor lady gave. Apparently her grandson brought some in to help give her a boost with her mobility during the day. What a helpful man!

## Sleep Deprivation: It is better to be tired than wired:

A few years ago, the popular US TV series MythBusters had two candidates stay awake all night in order to perform complex tasks in the morning. Interestingly, sleep deprivation above 21 hours is similar to drinking up to the legal limit of 0.08% (80mg per 100ml blood - UK) (31). Anyway, one candidate had to consume a lot of energy drinks and coffee and the other had to abstain totally from caffeine. Not surprisingly, the one who consumed coffee and caffeinated energy drinks failed most of the aptitude tests, including driving skills, the card game of snap and physical agility and balance tests. The 'caffeine man' was so fired-up that he was too quick (with snap) or too neurotic with the driving (there were a lot of scary distractions) and he was all over the place with the balance tests. So, MythBusters concluded that it is better to be tired than wired. There you have it.

# CHAPTER 8
# NIGHTSHIFTS

Are referred to as the **graveyard shift** because years ago people were sometimes unintentionally buried alive, so in 1829 Dr Taberger invented a system that placed a piece of string on the hands, head and feet of a body that went up a drainpipe-like tunnel that was attached to a bell on a stick above ground. A bell-housing prevented it from ringing accidently by perching birds. Those performing cemetery upkeep would keep an ear out during the day whilst working, but from dusk to dawn it was someone's sole job to listen out for any bells that may be rang at night, hence the term 'graveyard shift' (32). As a nurse, I've seen a lot of dead people and I cannot imagine mistaking someone alive as being dead. Still, Juliet fooled Romeo so it's potentially possible.

When doing nightshifts, the daily sunshine enjoyed by so many has been my true nemesis: the Achilles heel of the nightshift worker. Nightshifts have long been documented as being bad for your overall health, with some even suggesting that working nights may well lead to an early grave. I disagree, but then I refuse to come into alignment with a statement that could enforce an early demise.

So why *are* they so detrimental to our health? Well, hopefully we all know that they disturb the bodies circadian rhythm, which is the internal process that regulates our sleep-wake cycle, and the circadian rhythms (33) are also the mental, physical and behavioural changes that we experience within a 24-hour cycle. This is more commonly known as your *body clock*.

Mental health is definitely affected, even if the work area is not particularly stressful. Those who suffer from Seasonal Affective

Disorder (SAD, I know) may feel this more whilst working on nights, as less daylight is seen or enjoyed. I soon realise how much I take sunshine and blue sky for granted when I've started a season of nights again. And how the morning sun seems so tempting to stay awake and enjoy post-shift, but I know that I'll be knackered for that night if I do.

Never done nightshifts before? Try camping out and not going to sleep for a whole night, or go on an international night flight and stay awake. You may find that you display the characteristics of nervousness, irritability and anxiety, or that you're simply just sleepy and grumpy but I'll stop naming dwarves now. Once you've arrived at your destination and hotel room, note how you dealt with other people along the way. Were you restrained and both polite and pleasant to everyone? Now take that groggy feeling and imagine having to help an elderly person who has been doubly incontinent and is now wandering about in their room refusing to be cleaned or changed. Now you've got some insight to how nurses and care-workers have to behave under some *unique and interesting* circumstances, so please be nice to them.

Experts recommend 7-9 hours of quality sleep each night for adults to achieve optimal health. Night workers who get this amount are pretty rare. It could be argued that it is the lack of sleep rather than actually working at night that causes the health issues, but I won't split hairs trying to get this thesis cemented into the British Medical Journal hall of fame.

According to a 2012 study by the BMJ, working nights also increases the risk of developing diabetes, heart disease and obesity (34). The suppression of melatonin and the general discombobulation of other regulatory hormones probably has more of a detrimental effect than has been documented, and just because an individual feels okay doesn't mean that their internal homeostasis is in balance. Other studies show that eating at night impairs the body's ability to process sugar or glucose, as the hormone leptin is affected by sleep disruption.

Many a 'cuddly' nightshift worker has said that they put all their weight on whilst working nights. Those evil and manipulative nightshifts are apparently the sole reason why Pam went from a size 10 to a size 18. However, I have a different theory having done agency nursing on and off for many years, and have worked in pretty much all healthcare settings as I have seen a phenomenon that crosses all races, cultures, languages, religions and genders, and that is the responsibility of self-control.

The cakes, biscuits, chocolates etc., do become hard to resist at 2am when I'm sleep deprived, so I can see how people pack on weight working nights. I'm not being mean, but from observation it is usually the chunky person who has their hands in the cookie jar the most. Try putting a box of chocolates in a staffroom and watch who attacks them the hardest. The same person will then say that they can't seem to lose weight, whilst packing on an extra 500cals/night for that confection injection.

Now I get that some people have genuine hormonal or genetic predispositions to obesity, but it's interesting to note that nearly every overweight person thinks that it's them, and statistically, it isn't. I challenge everyone to keep a food diary for a week, with everything that you eat and drink being charted and have a look at the end. Enjoy the results; it will reveal what it reveals. You *can* lose weight on nightshifts, I know, because I have, and I have little to lose. However, you have to want it enough, SO set your face like flint to become a better you. I have every admiration for anyone who starts making small steps and lifestyle changes. It could be you…

The reality is that nightshifts lead to tiredness and fatigue, and this brings out the weaknesses in us all. Many times have I scoffed all my food by 2am and by 5am I'm on the scrounge, looking for a mini packet of wrapped biscuits (in the posh care homes) or the budget biscuit selection thrown into an old ice-cream tub. By 6am I'd no longer care whose hands have touched them, so I take one anyway and promise myself to either bring more food in or ration it next time.

On a nightshift everything gets exacerbated; smokers will smoke more, eaters will eat more, gossipers or wafflers won't leave you alone. Fatigue surely brings out the best in all of us! When I was a tradesman I remember the story of some men who were working too many days in a row and were so exhausted that one of them absolutely freaked out over a screw that was left on the floor and he really lost his spit. Thankfully, they all realised that it was down to everyone's extreme fatigue, gave a 'thumbs-up' to the contractor, took some time off and got some rest.

Observation shows that most nightshift workers operate on their own 'reward system'. Meaning that they'll do a bit of work, or wait a couple of hours and then either eat something or go out for a smoke. Again, this is cross-cultural, gender, race etc., as people use this coping strategy to get through the night. I'm an Englishman, so I favour a nice cup of tea.

Regarding eating, after the first night, I simply switched to day/night reversal with the hours. Most care home shifts are 8-8, so I'd eat my breakfast before the shift, then I'd eat my main meal (good old sandwiches) at about 1am and then eat when I got home before bed at about 9am. I'll usually have an omelette, as it's high protein, plus cholesterol to help with testosterone production whilst I sleep, and it's low in carbs, cheap and quick to make. A real winner, but by day four I'm ready for a change.

I reverse the clocks with sleeping as well. I'd be in bed before 10am and not set my alarm until 5pm (sometimes 6pm) to try and get as much sleep as possible. On my last night I'd still go to bed before 10am but get up at 4pm, then stay awake until about 11pm and sleep through until the following morning. Weirdly, after my first nightshift on, having been awake for over 24 hours then I'd be lucky to stay asleep after 3pm, meaning little more than 5 hours, having been awake for over 24. It's tough, but it is what it is. After my last night I'd set my alarm for 4pm, get up, and then potter about until about 11pm and then return to bed and try to return to 'day mode'. I'm usually so tired after 4 nights with the workload, commuting, sleep loss etc., that I rarely wake before 6am anyway, so equilibrium almost restored.

I know a giant 125kg Hungarian hulk whom I'll refer to as AK47 who after working 4-6 nights will not go to sleep after his last one and stay awake all day, and maybe go into town. He's lucky that no-one irritated him in town otherwise he'd have taken their head off.

## Top Tips For Sleeping During The Day

- Avoid caffeine after midnight, particularly coffee. Tea has less caffeine and is less associated with the 'pick me up' feeling of coffee. I have my tea black, therefore it is brewed weaker than regular tea, so I consume it up until about 5am whilst on nights. The problem with caffeine is that it stays in your system for hours after you feel the effects, so it can prevent you from sleeping well after work.

- Drink water whenever possible to avoid the problems caused by caffeine.

- Nap when possible whilst on your break. Even just closing your eyes in a busy staff room and letting your mind switch off for five minutes is beneficial.

- Get sunlight pre/post shift even for just a minute or two, and/or consider vit D supplements.

- Alcohol can make you fall asleep faster, but it also reduces rapid-eye-movement (REM) sleep, being the restorative phase of your sleep cycle, therefore you interfere with your body's ability to repair itself. That said, I've had great results with a large neat vodka/whisky/rum before I hit the pillow. I'm buzzing after a nightshift as I'm overtired, and the alcohol helps me to wind down quickly without filling me with fluid (beer/wine). That's just a shot or three, not half a bottle.

- Sleep in the best environment that you can make, keeping the room at the ideal temperature for you, keep it dark, use eyepatch and earplugs if required, switch off WIFI and put your phone onto flight mode.

- In summertime, try to leave windows open at night before you go to work, that way your home will be cooler for when you go to bed in the morning.

Most shift-workers do end up with some form of sleep debt, and must try, where possible to repay this with adequate sleep on days off or at least, by living as healthy a lifestyle as possible.

**Point to Ponder:** Since you have been proactive enough to buy this book then you are obviously self-aware and teachable. Perhaps you could consider an online side-hustle which could generate an income that could, in time, allow you to reduce or even quit your nightshifts altogether. Have a think about it…

# BASIC SLEEP ACCESSORIES

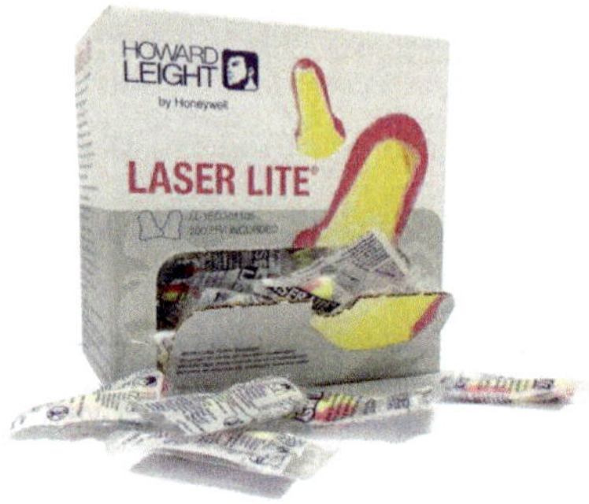


**Ear plugs:** The standard conical or straight cylindrical plugs didn't work for me, nor did the mouldable wax ones either. Between them all they either fell out, went in too far, didn't cancel noise sufficiently or irritated my ears. Then there are the silicon ones that look like a Zoom rocket ice-lolly (but smaller, warmer and in a uniform colour), but the 'stick' can catch on the pillow case and either get pulled out completely or just disturb my sleep.

Thankfully my ear plug conundrum came in the form of these Laser Lite ear plugs, which block up to 35dB. They are made of foam, and individually wrapped for hygiene purposes; what a blessing they were when I finally discovered them. One's ear plug journey cannot be underestimated, and mine is now complete. Yes I do wear them for more than one sleep, and the packet that they come in is the perfect storage envelope until their next use. However, when I go past several sleeps (it's variable; one to four) then my ears will itch when the plugs are inserted again, so I pop a new pair in. All I know is that I get several sleeps out of them and then they get binned. They are available on eBay in various packet sizes if you just want to try a few before buying a box of 200 pairs.

**Eye masks**

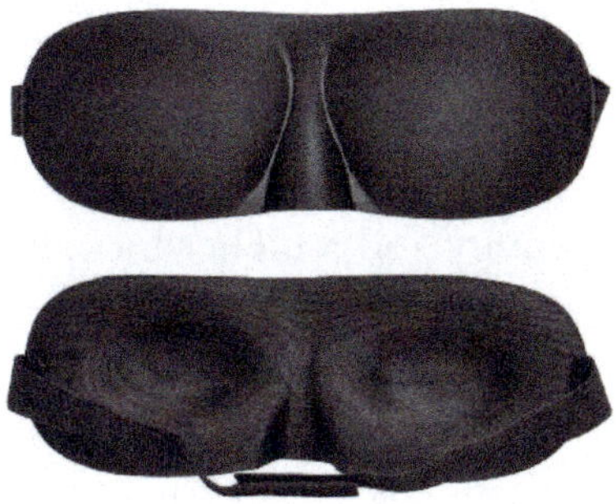

Are those ones that you get on flights okay to use? The short answer is yes, but there are much better versions available. Generally, standard eye masks are priced between £1-£10 respectively, but luxury ones can go higher than £100.

These are the 3-D masks that look like a mini padded bra and are supposed to be better as they keep the fabric off your eyelids. Try to avoid ones with a Velcro strap (like the ones pictured) to avoid hair pulling.

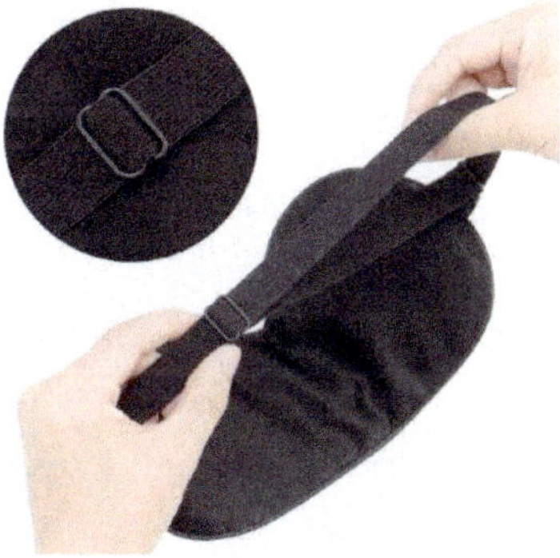

I've managed perfectly well with this type of eye mask, adjustable to avoid excessive pressure, and they keep the light out perfectly. Made of silk with a cotton liner, they wash well (I wash mine in the shower) and are less than £10 off eBay.

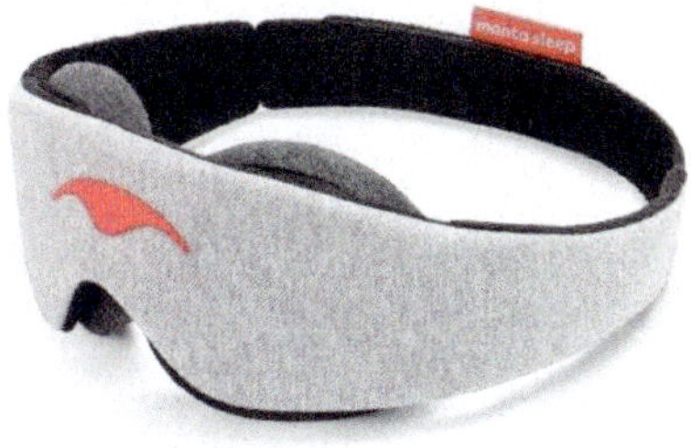

The Manta sleep mask seems to be the epitome of quality and design, with circular foam pads that wrap around your eyes. Their sales pitch is that having a sleep mask pressed against your eyes causes blurred vision due to corneal distortion, plus a reduction in circulation.

The Manta starts from about $35 up to $150, and yes, I get that this is a lot of money, but if you think of airline pilots, entrepreneurs, and those travelling business class everywhere then it's a small price to pay for what could result in more productivity and a higher income due to having better quality sleep.

When wearing an eye mask, there is a greater potential to develop a stye, which is caused by a blockage of one of the oil glands in the eyelids. This allows bacteria to grow inside the blocked gland. Not good. Styes are generally not contagious, but if you're prone to oily skin then you may be more susceptible to styes whilst wearing an eye mask.

**TOP-TIPS:**

- Avoid the free flight masks or any from the pound shop. They are cheap, non-adjustable, usually too tight and are made of polyester which can get very hot and sweaty in summer.
- Velcro type fastenings may get caught in your hair or on the pillow as you turn over and come undone and/or wake you up, and non-adjustable elastic straps can put too much pressure on your face, causing discomfort.
- Silk is comfortable and affordable.
- Try several inexpensive ones, and when you've found a style that you like then buy a few more. Keep one in your glove compartment of your car (along with a toothbrush and a set of ear plugs) as this enables you to stay over at a friend's house if you've had one too many and at least get a reasonable night's sleep there. Also, leave one at home when you go

on holiday; that way, if anything happens to your luggage en-route back then you'll still be okay when you get home.

**A word of caution**: you may become so reliant on one of these that you find that you can't sleep without one, even if your room is pitch black. I had to wean myself off them as I became addicted to the sensation and the habit, and then really struggled to sleep without one, so be warned. That said, when I do a block of night shifts I always use them.

**FUN FACT:** Eyelash mites are present on 23-100% of adults (35), and are particularly prevalent in the elderly. I finally got to experience them myself from an unknown source, likely work-related. They're not too bad, like a tingling sensation around the base of the eyelash, but I decided to part company with them. I didn't fancy tea-tree oil near my eyeballs, nor my local pharmacy or GP, so I went online and read about using coconut oil. The theory being after you've smeared your eyes with the coconut oil the demodex mites suffocate and die. My next day off I mauled the oil panda-style around my eyes, watched a film (reading was a bit too blurry), showered later and all good; no more itching. Cleared with one application. Happy days.

# CHAPTER 9
# TECHNOLOGY & GADGETS

James Bond saves the world with them, teenagers love them, and many seniors hate them. The rise of technology is ubiquitous in our modern world. As we can't avoid it, let's have a look at a few gadgets that could prove a worthy alternative to counting sheep.

**Luxe 750DAB**

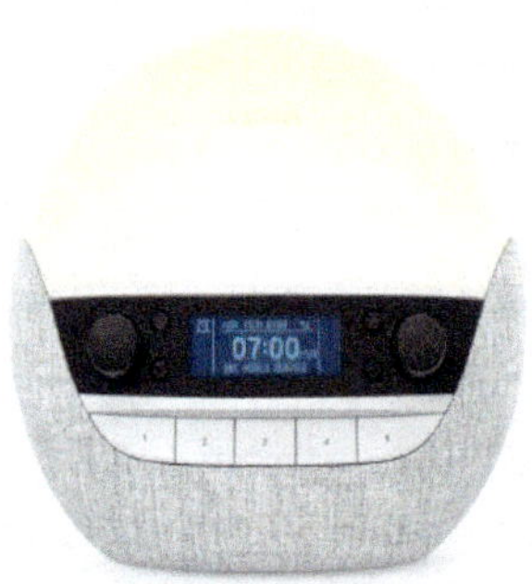


The main aim of this product is that it has a reducing light that is programmable for night, and a steadily increasing light for the morning, to allow you to wake up 'naturally' rather than using that poxy rooster alarm on your phone.

The review of this product according to T3 is as follows:

*'The wake up light and sunset functions are genuinely lovely on the Luxe 750DAB, but convoluted settings and navigation make the experience more stressful than it should be. Bluetooth connectivity means it's handy to use as a speaker but the DAB radio function here is limited by location and requires the 60cm aerial to be fully extended.'*

So, the pros of buying the Luxe 750DAB is that the wake-up light provides an excellent sunset function which can be a gamechanger. There is a good selection of sounds and it has a USB charger on the back.

The cons are that it can be quite fiddly to set-up, the DAB has a limited range and the aerial has to be fully extended for the radio to function. The cost is a bit prohibitive at an average of £200.

**Philips Sleep and Wake-up Light with Relax Breathe**

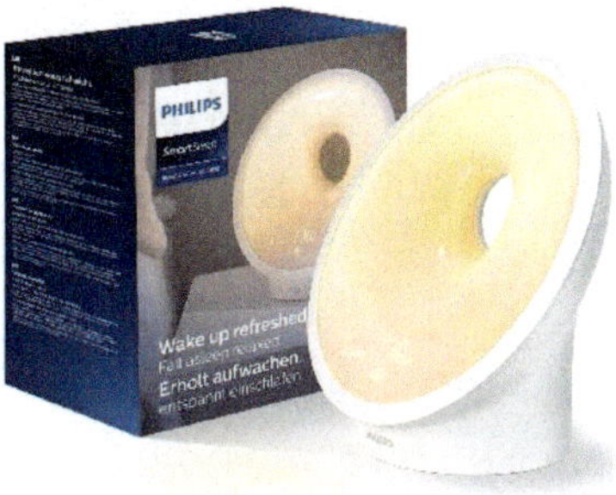


This gadget is clinically proven to improve general wellbeing after waking, with 92% of users finding it easier to get up in the morning with this device.

It offers a feature called 'Relax Breathe', which is a light-guided wind-down breathing system that helps you relax to sleep while the sunset simulation is preparing your body for sleep. It features a smart touch display for easier device control. There are personalised brightness levels to choose which one is right for you. Product dimensions (W x D x H): 225x220x120 mm. Philips have a wide range of these devices, the more features, the higher the price, starting from about £70. One reviewer claimed to work in the lighting industry and he recommended Philips above other brands due the quality of the light, having tried several others before.

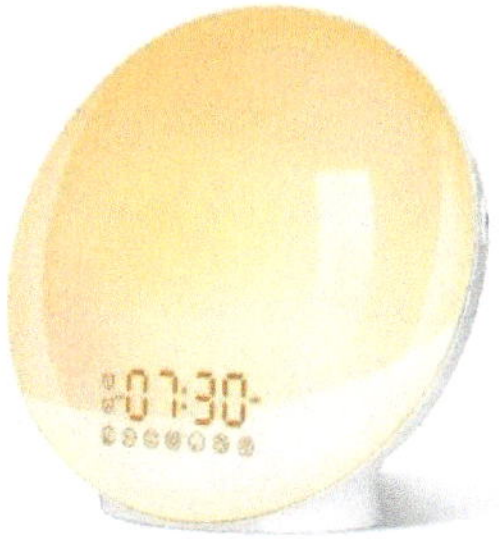


A cheaper alternative would be a simple sunrise/sunset alarm clock. It may not have a radio facility nor a USB charger, but if you like listening to the radio then chances are that you have one already, and if not then nothing lost. Available from Amazon for about £30, it's a good entry level choice to see if you like using light to assist with your sleep, and can always be given away to parents with young children as a 'don't leave your room until the colour changes' sleep training device.

**Bose Sleepbuds 2**

Bose needs no introduction for its quality of sound across a wide range of products. The Sleepbuds 2 are designed to mask sound to help you to drop off to sleep. If you choose white noise, instrumentals or natural sounds such as rainforests or ocean swells then you may be more likely to drift off to sleep. Soothing noises can help those with tinnitus, as silence can really intensify the ringing/buzzing noises; I know, it does. These earbuds are non-bulky and so allow for side sleep.

With most technology it takes time to load music onto them, and they have Bluetooth, which can still be used if your phone is on flight mode. You will still be able to hear a doorbell as they mask sound but don't totally block it. They also have an alarm function on them.

**Kokoon Ear Buds**

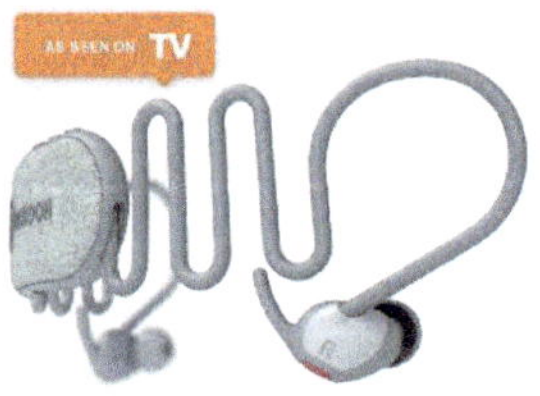


These tiny, soft earbuds are perfect for side sleepers as they sit snugly in the ear. The audio has a function that auto-fades as you drift off. There is also an optional white noise function to mask disturbances. There are sleep-monitoring sensors that can provide data to assist in a better night's sleep in the future. As per the photo they have been featured on TV and have come up in several top 10 searches for sleep gadgets.

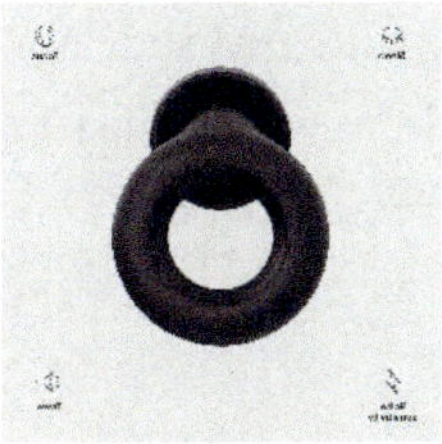

A cheaper alternative would be Loop Quiet, and although they don't play any music, they are designed for noise reduction, boasting up to 27 decibels lower (although the Laser Lite plugs stop 35dB). They are made of soft silicone, come in a range of colours and have 4 different sizes per kit, meaning a total of 8 pieces, thus enabling you to make the perfect size choice if/when replacements are required. They are designed for a variety of uses, including concerts, workplace noise and studying, as well as sleep, and should stay in place throughout the night.

**Withings Sleep Analyser**

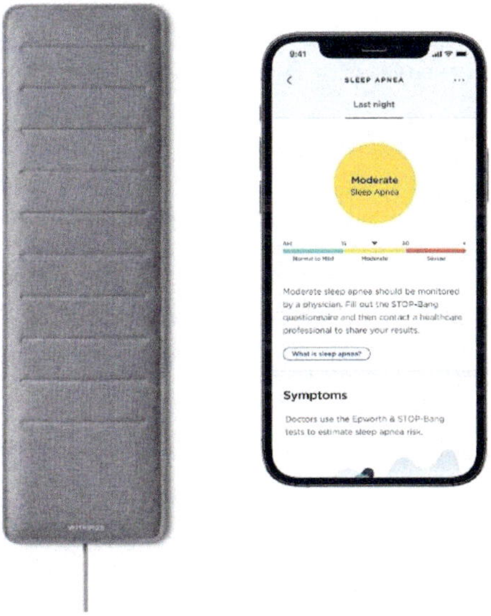


This is a 25"x7.5" (63x19cm) pad that is plugged in and inserted under your mattress at chest level.

The positive features are that it's non-wearable, therefore your sleep will be uninhibited by the device. Their website claims that it'll give you sleep-lab type results at home. Your sleep diaries will be pretty comprehensive, including average sleep durations for weekday/weekends, bedtime and wake-up times, snoring/breathing statistics, average heart rate and a visual representation of the time that you spent in bed, time spent asleep, and any extended times out of bed. You can also customise the time period of analysis, so if you are making lifestyle changes then you can monitor pre and post changes.

The disadvantage is that synching can take quite a while and that it's not particularly accurate for naps. It also wouldn't be ideal for nightshift workers due to the ongoing day/night reversal between blocks of shifts.

**Dreampad Pillow**

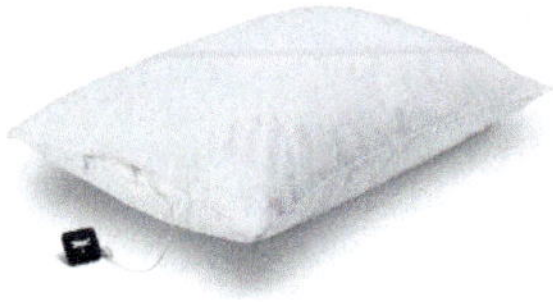

The pillows come in either memory foam or polyester, and work by attaching your smartphone and using the Dreampad app. These pillows are very good for those who suffer with tinnitus, or for those whose partners snore, or for those who simply want to unwind and drift off with soothing music. The main advantage is that the sounds can only be heard by the person using the pillow.

**Somnox Pillow**

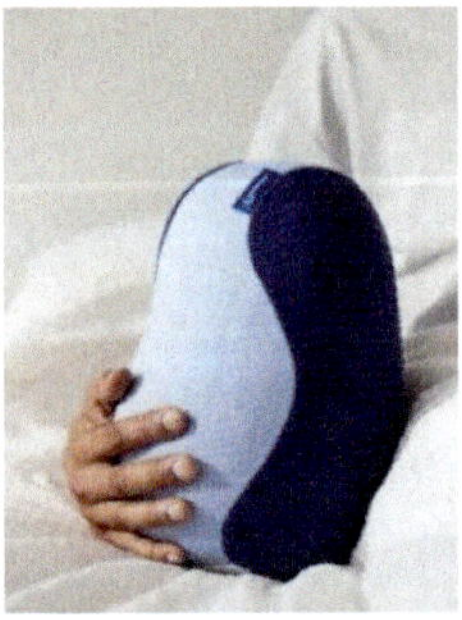

This is essentially a teddy bear's body to cuddle, but it has rave reviews due to its rising and falling movements that mimic breathing. The 'breathing' is set to a slow pace, allowing the user to relax and settle their body. They boast the ability to fall asleep, stay asleep and return to sleep if woken in the night. A real comforter.

**Dodow**

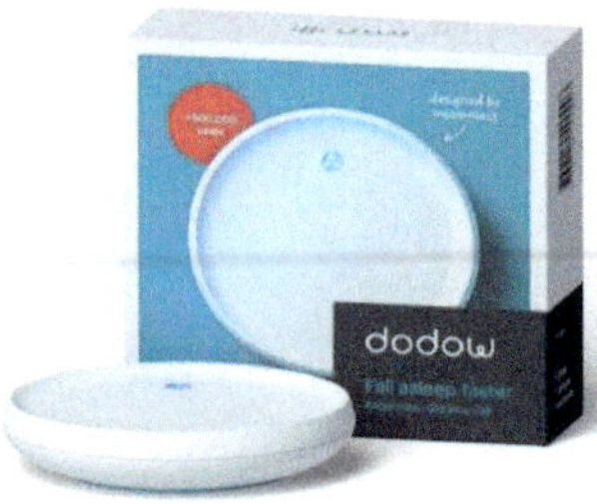


This is basically a light generating machine that you can sync your breathing to which then relaxes and leads to sleep. Inhale when the light expands, exhale when the light retracts. The exhalation light is slightly longer to create a sense of tiredness, therefore helping you fall asleep. There is an 8 minute and a 20-minute mode setting. It will then switch itself off.

**BedJet 3 Dual Zone Climate Comfort Sleep System for Couples**

This system works like the hospital air blankets used for patients who

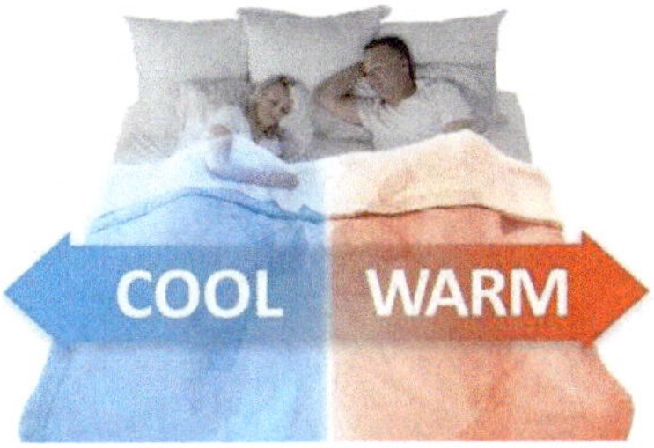


are hypothermic or are coming out of theatres post-op. Quicker at warming than an electric blanket, they have the ability to dry sweat due to the air circulating. As the picture suggests, it can be on a hot or cold setting depending on your preference, and both hot and cold can be on at the same time. For those with significant temperature differences or issues this could be a game-changer!

**Netatmo Indoor Air Quality Monitor**

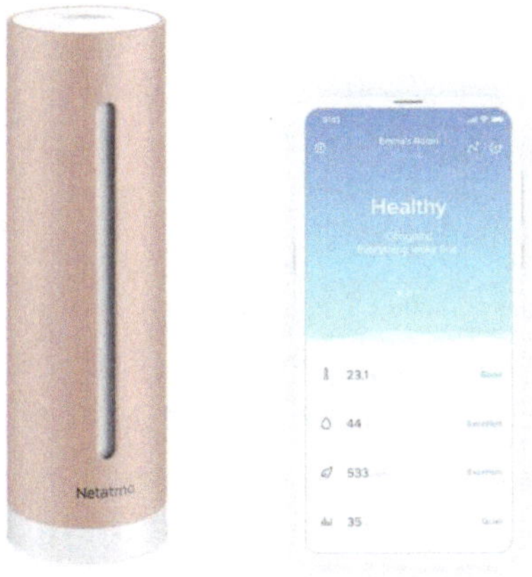


This device monitors the air quality and humidity, but also noise and the room temperature as well. It'll make suggestions via your smartphone when it detects something out of its ranges and then notify you.

I could see many parents having them in young children's bedrooms.

**Sleepace**

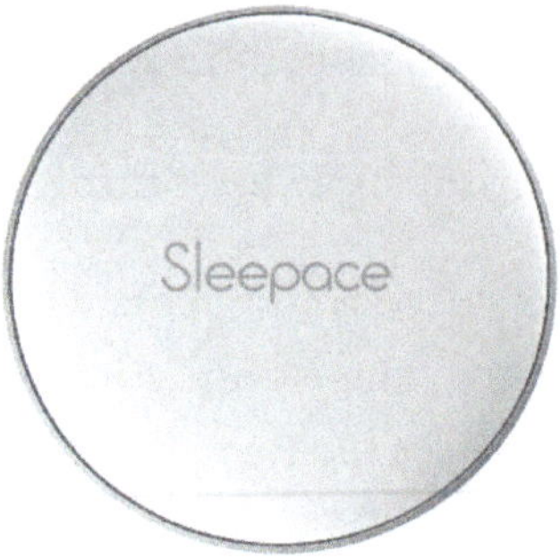


Only about 3.5cm, or 1.5" and it clips onto the pillow case. At under £20 it is a good entry level for monitoring your sleep data.

**Fitbit Watch**

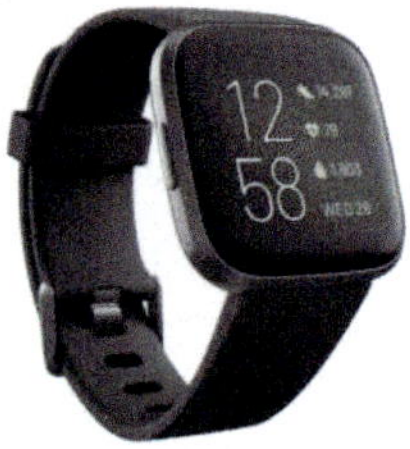


These are under £90 in Argos UK. Most people are familiar with the Fitbit; if not, find someone who has one and ask them. Word of mouth is better than any online review anyway. They have the usual cardiac functions to monitor heartrate in relation to sleeping patterns, so if you can handle sleeping with a watch, then this could be the best all-rounder watch to have, as there is lots of biofeedback to analyse.

**Oura Ring**

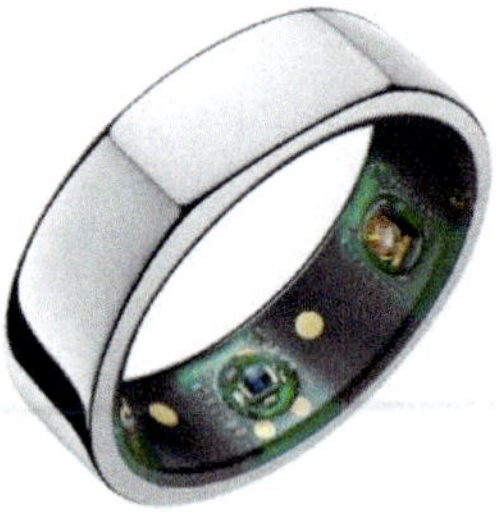

Wake up to in-depth analysis about your deep sleep, light sleep, REM sleep, blood oxygen levels, and more. They boast the largest amount of sleep biofeedback and have many positive reviews. The great thing is that it monitors your body and sleep whilst being in direct contact, yet it's small enough not to interfere with your sleep.

It tracks calorie burn, counts steps and hourly movement, including your elevated activity and workout intensity based on your heart rate. It is also water, sweat, hand cream and soap-proof.

It only needs to be charged every five days for about an hour.

At about $300-$350 it's not cheap, but it does look good, with four colours to choose from, and the fact that it can be worn unobtrusively all the time is a big plus. It can also replace calorie counters, heart rate monitors and pedometers, so it really is quite a concise bit of kit. The data appears to be displayed well, via your smart screen. There is a $5.99/month membership fee, but if this lapses then you still get the sleep, readiness, and activity features. Check out their website, it's pretty simple to follow.

**Calm App**

This app provides meditations for a variety of different situations, but also offers music, soundscapes and sleep stories. Stories, you might ask? Think of David Attenborough's soothing and melodic voice narrating some form of nature programme, and how soporific his dulcet tones are. Think of the stories that you (hopefully) heard as a child, yet the adult versions are intentionally far more boring, such as travelling tales that add all the incidentals along the way. These allow your mind to pause and sigh with a restful 'aaah' as you lie back and drift off. You can add the stories to your phone or stream to headphones or speakers.

The free content is always enticing, but insufficient to last an adequate amount of time, cue the subscription. The Premium service is £39.99 for the year BUT you do get a free 7-day trial. A lifetime subscription costs £399.99 or equivalent of 10 years' subscription in simple terms (priced in June 2023). Give it a whirl for 7 days, the website does look good and is simple to use.

**Gadget disclaimer**: *it is generally advisable to consult a healthcare professional before investing or using any form of sleep gadget. I'm not entirely sure why, but safety is our number one priority…*

A section of electronic gizmos and gadgets wouldn't be complete without a tribute to the good old Teasmade. Remember those? They were generally cream-coloured, which was partly due to there being over 50 shades of beige in the 1970s, and also because most things white quickly ended up beige anyway from the hazy fumes of cigarette smoke that settled throughout the home.

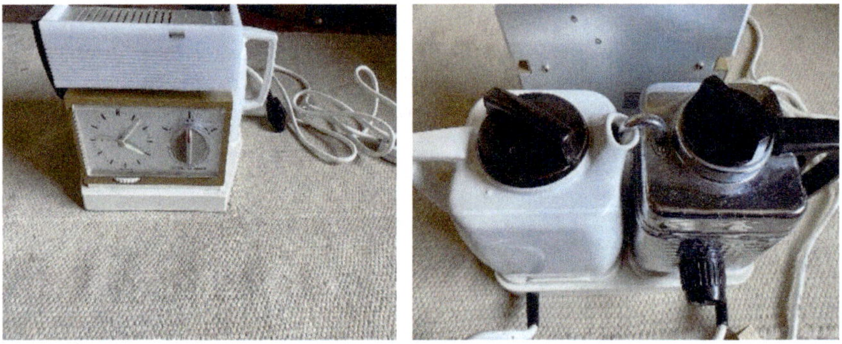

*Pictured above is a Goblin Teasmade, complete with an alarm guaranteed to wake you up to a hot cup of Maxwell House or a mug of Mellow Birds as Mellow Birds will make you smile…*

# CHAPTER 10
# WINDING DOWN

**Sleep-hygiene** is the buzz-word for the preparation and practices that you perform to get a good night's sleep. The books and the experts like to tell us what to do, how to do it and when to do it, but I don't. This book is about suggestions that you can do that will fit in with your lifestyle, because we don't all live in cosy sound-proof apartments. Some of us live in studio flats, tiny houses or yurts, some share with too many others, some live in a van to surf every day, some are unlucky enough just to sofa-surf. Whatever your *current* situation, you can still improve your sleep. Everything is temporary, some of us need to be reminded of this.

Books and articles mention 'proper sleep-hygiene' yet they offer a *one size fits all* solution.

Good sleep habits are important to your overall health, and for those around you. Think about your daily schedule and how this can be improved. Your nutrition and fluids consumed, physical activities and evening routines. This may be different from one day to the next, particularly with shift-workers.

You know how your body works, or at least you should by now. Aristotle was right when he said (along with Plato & Socrates) *'Know Thyself'*. If you don't feel well enough rested in the morning then you probably need to evaluate your sleep. Ditto if you're not getting seven or more hours of sleep per night or you're sleepy throughout the day. That said, remember the variables. Not everyone is a morning person, so you may feel groggy upon waking. If you're busting it out at the gym and over 40 then you'll probably feel tired/achey the next day anyway and yet you might be genetically gifted and only need six hours per night.

Discuss winding down together, whether there is to be a TV in the bedroom, or whether children or pets sleep in your bed, snoring issues, room temperature and how you address arguments before bed (those fight or flight hormones will churn you up and make sleep pretty elusive unless resolved in some way). Some ancient wisdom advises not to let the sun go down on your anger, so do try to resolve conflict before your head hits the pillow. Don't assume that you know your partner's preferences or needs, and definitely don't assume that they know yours, because unless you've told them, they won't. Communication is key.

Sleep experts seem to emphasise the need to keep a consistent sleep schedule that can be adhered to every day. Such experts haven't considered shift-workers whilst they sit in their ivory towers though. Establishing a routine is desirable, and can be very beneficial, but you still need to live a little, so tweak it and be spontaneous from time to time. I've had to deal with issues using my phone, then the obligatory doomscrolling that followed meant that I switched my phone off just ten minutes before lights-out and still had a great night's sleep. I've also switched my phone off an hour before bed (plus laptop, TV etc) and had a poor night's sleep. A good night's sleep is not a cut-and-dried, black and white affair. There will always be variables, but establishing good habits remains beneficial even if consistency is a problem.

Avoid getting into bed unless ready for sleep; for example, don't head to bed earlier to doomscroll on your phone.

- Limit bed use to sleeping and sex.
- Set up your environment for success (i.e., cool, dark room, proper bedding, etc.).

- Limit or avoid stimulating substances including nicotine, caffeine, and alcohol (especially later in the day).
- Avoid looking at screens too close to bedtime (i.e., turn off electronics 30 minutes to an hour before bedtime) ideally. This is a tough one and does require self-discipline.
- Limit the amount of food and type of food consumed a few hours before bedtime (i.e., don't eat a large (or spicy) meal or fill up on heavy, processed snacks right before trying to sleep).
- Make a bedtime routine in the hour before trying to sleep (i.e., take a hot bath, wash your face, meditate, or listen to a sleep story).
- Limit naps to 20 minutes if possible.
- Get an adequate amount of physical activity.

## SUPPER & ALL THINGS FOOD

There is an old saying of; eat the breakfast of a king, the lunch of a prince and the dinner of a pauper. However, many have moved on from three squares a day, and there are SO many different options available, so do what works for you. Obviously you know your body and how it functions, but the old adage of not eating a heavy meal late in the evening is a good one, especially rich or spicy foods as your liver will have to process them and your sleep may well be lighter as a result. Your liver is engaged in many activities and the energy it creates warms the blood that passes through it. Hence the night sweats after a bender and the shivers when fasting for several days.

I went for several years whereby I would have a banana within reach so that if I wake up hungry at 2am then I don't need to move to eat and I don't need to put the light on either. A cereal bar is a better alternative, as it can be kept in your bedside cabinet. That said, 2am munchies can become addictive, so I had to wean myself off this as it had begun to form part of my nightly routine. I really had to trick my mind into believing that I wasn't hungry when I woke up at 2am and therefore didn't need to eat.

Along with the benefit of regular exercise (a physically-demanding job counts), we all know that eating a balanced diet is the best for our overall health. Getting the amino acid tryptophan, which helps to regulate sleep, will benefit. Foods high in tryptophan include turkey, chicken, cheese, milk, cottage cheese, egg whites, fish, peanuts, plus sunflower and pumpkin seeds. Stress and anxiety can be very taxing for your muscles, and this is where magnesium is beneficial, but most of us don't really get enough (see Chemical Cosh chapter). It is found in wholegrains, dark-green, leafy vegetables, and low-fat milk and yoghurt, plus soybeans, baked beans, lentils, and nuts, such as peanuts, almonds and cashews.

Bananas are the sleep wonder food because they contain magnesium, potassium AND tryptophan, which is converted into serotonin and melatonin (36). Try combining one with some yoghurt and berries whilst you reflect and unwind instead of reaching for a tub of ice-cream. Oily fish such as salmon, trout, mackerel and sardines contain high volumes of vitamin B6 which helps the body to produce melatonin. Dates are also a good source of melatonin.

Monitor your fluid intake in the evening. That last cup of tea might not be a great idea if you are prone to getting up in the middle of the night to pass urine (medically known as nocturia). I thought that I drank nearer to 3 litres of fluid per day, so whilst writing this I did a simple fluid chart, and was shocked to discover that in 3 days I was between 4.5-5.5 litres per day. Gosh, no wonder I kept needing that 'last minute wee' before falling asleep. I've reduced my fluids to approximately 3 litres and feel better for it. Perhaps my electrolytes were a bit off? Anyway, you're probably not drinking enough WATER, so try the fluid chart for yourself, as most people don't seem to drink enough, something I have always found very strange. I aim to get the majority of fluid down me before teatime, and after 7pm I sip more water as I start to be on fluid wind down from then. I'm not retentive about it, I still have a life, but I'm just more self-aware than I was, because I want less bladder action at night.

Chamomile tea is a bit of a wonder-tea as it has anti-inflammatory properties, soothes cold symptoms, is good for your heart (research ongoing), helps with digestion, anxiety and sleep. It soothes sore throats, and is good for your immune system. I'll frequently, but not daily, have an evening tisane, whether it be a chamomile or other herbal tea, or sometimes a weak, black Earl Grey, usually from a cup and saucer like the jolly Englishman that I am.

## BATHING

To get clean before going to bed or when one wakes in the morning is both a personal and occupational choice. Hopefully no mechanics go to bed without getting clean beforehand. Some people can go a few days without smelling at all, some can't even manage a few hours. It is what it is, we are what we are. The good old experts claim that having a hot bath before bed lowers *core* temperature which helps people fall asleep more quickly. The only way that I could see that happening logically is if the bather then parades around in their underwear because they are too hot from the bath, and they therefore cool down by default. Yet other experts say that having a hot shower right before bed can disrupt your sleep due to being too hot. A hot bath makes me hotter all over. Who would have thought that? I'm not an expert. Do what you enjoy, but having a good old soak in the tub will relax your muscles better than having a shower.

Not so many people like a cold shower in the morning, but for sheer self-control, grit your teeth type of determination, they do work. There is a sense of euphoria afterwards, plus a sense of achievement that can really set the rest of the day in motion. Try it, cold is cold for everyone, so it's a real leveller, and it's well documented as having numerous health benefits. Just ask Wim Hof.

## EXERCISE

You don't need to be told that exercising for 20+ minutes per day will improve your overall health, and a lot of research points towards doing exercise in the morning to ensure a better night's sleep. Do what you can, when and where you can. When I was in poor health I used to do standing push-ups holding onto the kitchen counter and bodyweight squats holding onto a chair, whilst the kettle boiled. Exercise can be done at home with no kit even as an absolute beginner or if you're very out of shape. I've done killer workouts and been in bed within an hour and slept well. I've also done them early evening and still been all 'revved up' at bedtime and unable to wind down. Ditto hot baths, cold showers etc., so is it the exercise or the mindset?

You probably all know your chronotype, of being either an early bird or a night owl, but such labels are not an exact science; we all have variables, plus our employment doesn't always allow us to work out at a time that would be the most favourable. Even though I'm a morning person, the thought of a morning workout is incredible unappealing, so this usually happens at home whilst my dinner is cooking. If exercise is done in the evening then 2-3 hours before bedtime is advisable. That said, like dieting, there are so many contributing factors to consider, including lifestyle, your goals, your body-type and what you actually term as exercise. Working out at home, doing a very simple routine of push-ups, pull-ups, sit-ups, some KB swings can really help to build muscle or tone the body. However, it's unlikely to get the heart (or brain) racing as much as going to a gym and working out for an hour.

When I used to attend a gym I didn't factor in the stresses of travelling to the gym, the social interaction (just basic politeness) and all the external stimuli that goes hand in hand with being in a gym. Physically my pulse and resps returned to normal as soon as I got home, but I'll still be processing the experience for some time. The joys of being an overthinker! And seeing men twice my size being alpha-jerks. And seeing women in tight clothes. Aaargh!! Then I discovered callisthenics and primal movements and have not returned to a gym.

Goals are good, and that elusive 'beach body' is not a bad one to go for, because generally speaking, an attractive body is a healthy body. Get outside, get some fresh air, open windows, eat a bit less (generally) and move a bit more. It will do you good. We *all* have busy lifestyles, but if determined enough, we can *all* find a way to get outside a bit more. Whilst at work I've been on several 'virtual' smoke breaks outside, and the fresh air pressed the reset button in my mind and I returned far better than I left.

Exercise helps to relieve stress and it boosts the happy-feeling endorphins and serotonin, which assists with the function of sleeping. Exercise also helps with the production of adenosine, and is thought to help with melatonin release as well. However, it is fair to comment that exercising too late can also cause spikes in adrenaline and cortisol; both of which will prevent winding down quickly. But, if you know your body, your temperaments etc., then it may work well for you to exercise late, have a warm shower, and then crash. We all know that any type of exercise is better than none, but for some people it is the elephant in the room as to why they can't sleep, although exercise is by no means the panacea of insomnia. Shame. I'm certainly not going to prescribe or suggest an exercise routine here; just do what you can to move a bit more and get as much fresh air as possible alongside an exercise programme suited to your goals. Are you not sure about aligning your body into a pose that evokes the kundalini spirits of yoga to make Shiva happy? Try Pilates instead, or design your own stretching programme based on your limitations and goals, that way it's planned for YOUR needs.

There is a danger that we can over-think our chronotypes, jobs, body-types, workout goals, diet, insomnia etc., and wallow in the apathy of analysis-paralysis. Look at the military, and how they train, often doing sleep-deprived training exercises. They cut out all the fluff of variables and produce some pretty stacked individuals. How? By just getting on with it; reflect on that, quit the excuses and get out there. Not having a staff-sergeant barking out orders with the threat of a beasting may limit your determination levels but just give it your best shot each time.

## RELAXATIONAL BREATHING

Breathing is important, we all know that, but how many of us actually take the time to analyse or assess our own breathing? Most people view breathing like they view their own digestion system, in that they take it for granted as long as it works. This is a real shame, as, unlike digestion, we do have some control over our breathing. Sportspeople, dancers, singers etc., all know this, but the average person doesn't - and they should, as it can be very beneficial.

Ever taken a deep sigh for no apparent reason and felt instantly better? Chances are you were in a certain position physically, mentally, emotionally whereby your breathing was very shallow, and the sudden deep inhalation provided better blood oxygen levels, giving your brain a much-needed boost. But it's so much more than that. Sighing can bring relief to a particular feeling, or happen when we have either a heightened or lowered mood. Many researchers indicate that sighing is a negative thing (37). Personally, I disagree, as I have had some incredible releases of pent-up tension and frustration by simply taking a few really deep breaths which have triggered yawns, or randomly had a deep whimsical sigh and felt so much better. Not only does it boost my blood oxygen in the physical, but it releases all kinds of emotional tensions and releases dopamine and serotonin, both which help me to relax and feel better (38).

Many of us hold a lot of tension in our face and neck, especially when concentrating, so make a conscious effort to relax your tongue which is often pressing on the roof of your mouth. Check this for yourself, and if so, relax your tongue, puff your cheeks, scrunch your eyes and waggle your jaw; you may be surprised how tense you really were.

*The Iceman* Wim Hof's breathing method is worth checking out for most things breathing and for his cold-water achievements. So how do I make deep breathing/sighing into a breathwork exercise programme before bed? In short, I don't. The problem that I've found with any form of breathwork exercises is that I need to get so many things right: the location, time, listening to breathing rhythms, counting my breaths etc.

All that concentrating made me more tense, plus the dizziness, light-headedness and euphoria were not conducive to falling asleep. Breathing exercises known as the 4-4-8 or 4-7-8 method are supposed to help the individual fall asleep within two minutes. However, breathing in for 4 seconds, holding for 4 seconds and then breathing out for 6-8 seconds made me feel like I'd been swimming as I soon felt out-of-breath and dizzy. After about a minute of this 'relaxing exercise' I'd finally gasp for air like a free-diver surfacing after a personal best, so it didn't work for me.

Counting my resps is a truly Zen approach, but I was supposed to be relaxing, not concentrating. My own personal journey of faith means that I'm not comfortable with yoga and Hinduism nor harnessing Qi energy via Buddhism so I formed my own breathing method, as per 'the solution' below, and you can too.

**The Solution:** I'll take a few deep breaths between getting ready for, or climbing into bed. This usually triggers yawning or sighing, but not always. Sometimes a few deep breaths are enough. If I'm still a bit tense or stressed then I'll lie on my back with the lights off and breathe deeper but I'm not dogmatic about it. I usually tie this in with the 'Military Method' in the next section. Take deep 'belly-breaths', allowing your abdomen to rise and fall, and you can allow your mind to wander, as you're more likely to drift off, but try to keep your thoughts relaxational, which may take some discipline. Plan a breathing routine if you like, but for me, simplicity is key. I don't follow a plan and I don't deep breathe every night. I probably should, but there are a lot of things that I probably should be doing. I take a few deep breaths, have a yawn or two and call it a night.

## NAPS

It makes sense that adults need to be awake for about 16 hours in order to feel sleepy enough to get a full eight hours. This is why it is ideal (but not entirely practical) to awake and retire at roughly the same time every day, hence why naps are discouraged by most of the professionals, but not by me. Sometimes you might be absolutely hanging in the middle of the day, and a quick shut-eye from 5 mins to an hour may just do you the world of good.

The main advantages are:

- A short nap can help you to overcome sleepiness thereby increasing your alertness, especially if you didn't get enough sleep the night before.

- That brief sleep can enhance your cognitive abilities, by allowing your brain to rest and recuperate, and this can lead to an improved mental performance.

- Napping can help improve your mood and reduce feelings of irritability or stress. You get a break from your daily activities which can leave you feeling refreshed and rejuvenated.

- A well-timed nap can boost your productivity by restoring your focus and energy. They can help you recharge and maintain better performance throughout the day.

- Napping can also provide physical relaxation, reducing muscle tension and therefore helping you to feel more relaxed.

The main disadvantages are:

- If you nap for too long or wake up abruptly from a deep sleep stage, you may experience sleep inertia, whereby you wake up feeling groggy and disorientated. And grumpy. Your alertness may suffer and you'll be more tempted to reach for a caffeinated drink which may inhibit sleep later.

- Taking long or late-afternoon naps can interfere with your ability to fall asleep or stay asleep during the night. This can lead to difficulty establishing a regular sleep schedule and may contribute to insomnia.

- Regularly relying on naps may lead to dependency. It can also lead to a dysfunctional night's sleep, therefore creating excessive daytime tiredness which forms a vicious cycle. Naps may prevent your ability to address the root causes of your sleep issues.

- Few jobs will allow napping during the day, so they are likely to interfere with your work, study, or social life to some extent, even if you work from home.

Some people are refreshed by taking a nap, others get groggy and have their sleep pattern affected, so taking a nap depends on your lifestyle, needs and sleep patterns. It is always a good idea to set an alarm if you are concerned that you may oversleep. If napping improves your overall well-being without interfering with night-time sleep then go for it.

## MILITARY METHOD

The 'military method' of falling asleep has risen in popularity, partially due to its mystique, but also because it sounds too good to be true. As the name suggests it has been popularised by the US army and has been documented in Lloyd Bud Winter's 1981 book *Relax and Win: Championship Performance.* The technique was designed to help soldiers fall asleep quickly in any situation to allow for instant rest. This must have been particularly handy when sleeping in a platoon of 20+ soldiers back at the barracks.

The method is as follows:

1. Relax your entire face, including all your facial muscles and your tongue. You will be surprised how often you push your tongue against the roof of your mouth when stressed or concentrating. I pull all sorts of silly faces, frown and wiggle my jaw, which often sets off a yawn, which is much needed. Blow out your cheeks and then exhale. You were probably more tense than you thought!

2. Then rotate and drop your shoulders to release any tension and allow your hands to drop to the side of your body. Rotate your wrists and flex your hands. Visualising sun bathing or the safety of a canoe in the middle of a calm lake may work to help you relax.

3. Exhale, relaxing your body and focus on your breathing. Tense (or flex) your buttocks, thighs and calves and then relax them. The time held tense or the speed which you relax them doesn't matter. First tense, then relax after.

4. Now focus on clearing your mind for ten seconds, by imagining a relaxing scene. You've got to find something that works for you. Try speaking out, 'I'm so sleepy' or 'relax my

> mind' and repeating this for ten seconds, then continue repeating it in your mind. As you speak, so you become…

Experts and avid fans of this method say that you should fall asleep in about a minute or two after practice. True enough, by tensing and relaxing this does unwind the body which helps to activate the parasympathetic nervous system, which is responsible for our rest and recovery.

Statistics suggest that 96 percent of people who mastered this technique are able to fall asleep within two minutes of shutting their eyes. Personally, I doubt that, but it is the most effective when practised daily, and you should begin to reap the benefits after four to six weeks. I use this method when I've been busy and haven't had the time or am just too tired to do a stretching routine. This method does go some way to explaining the term 'military fatigues'.

## ELECTROMAGNETIC POLLUTION

Switch off your Wi-Fi if possible. This is so important. Your brain needs to unwind at night without unnecessary waves going through it. We can't stop TV waves and radio waves, but we can control home Wi-Fi to a certain extent. This may not make a difference, but it might. Research is sketchy, and of course WIFI and phone companies will tell you that your phone is safe to charge next to you and all will be well, but they don't mention potential radiation or sleep-wave disruption from charging. Unless it's in the small print that no-one reads.

TV, laptop, speakers, printers etc., all give off some form of EMF (electromagnetic frequency) when in use, and may well do when on standby, so I switch as many off as I can to avoid potential sleep interference. Unplug the landline and put your mobile phone on flight mode too. Do you really want a text at silly o'clock that gets your mind racing with excitement or dread? I've done this for years and unless I have to be on-call for work or a family crisis then tough luck if someone wants to contact me, I'll deal with it in the morning.

## ME TIME

We all like it, some people demand it as a right, some people sadly don't get enough of it, and everybody truly wants more of it. However, if you've not experienced your quota for the day then you may be tempted to stay up later to catch up with your social media which you will defend vehemently as 'trying to unwind'. I'm yet to find anything on Facebook or other social media platforms as 'unwinding' or relaxing. Moreover, I find that all forms of social media are at times, 'triggering' and I have, in the past, wasted hours of my life disagreeing with a random stranger who has an opposing opinion to myself about a particular subject, with both of us trying to prove the other one 'wrong'. What a waste of my time and emotions.

As for TikTok, Facebook reels, YouTube shorts or other sinkholes, we are entering into a world of wasted time. I was explaining to my teenage children that when you think that you should come off TikTok then the addiction called 'just one more' kicks in. The problem here is that if the video was rubbish then you'll have to finish on a good one. Several videos later and there is a cracking one, but to make up for all the rubbish, time-wasting videos that you've trawled through you'll watch just one more to finish on a high. The trouble is, the next one is disappointing, as is the next, and so you never really come off, or feel dissatisfied or cheated when you do. If this is in any way familiar to yourself then perhaps you need to evaluate how you spend your screen time.

I stopped watching TV about a decade ago, I do not have a licence and my TV is only plugged into a DVD player. The main reason is that I did not want to dedicate the next twenty+ years to keeping up to date with all the soaps, the Big Brother contestants, and the sheer meaninglessness of the celebrity award ceremonies. Besides, I don't like the annoying adverts. Remember that TikTok and other forms of social media, plus movies, anxiety-inducing shows, and/or video games are going to stimulate your brain and keep you awake. That said, I have gone down some fascinating and sometimes deeply distressing online rabbit holes as a 'truth-seeker' (friends call me a conspiracy-theorist) and have been captivated for hours. Perhaps only the Amish are immune to the trappings of tech?

A real danger is that you may be so exhausted that you start nodding off at about eight o'clock but you bravely stay up until 10pm in order to satiate your desire for 'me time'. Great, you achieved it, but your body and mind have not recovered as well as if you'd listened to your body, thrown in the towel at 8pm and been asleep just before 9pm. If you're falling asleep that early then your body needs it. Better to lose one night's 'me time' to rest and reset your body than to just keep going. The story rarely ends well for those who just keep going, hence the importance of knowing thyself, and getting adequate rest.

## THE SPIRITUAL BIT

*Woke Warning:* Those who don't believe that we are spiritual beings may want to skip this section.

If you are not at all religious and you are at the end of your rope with sleep loss then try crying out to the God that you don't believe in. Tell Him everything; at least you'll feel better for it afterwards.

You may also be interested to know that the Bible has quite a few references to sleep; you may not, but try declaring them out loud anyway. You may be surprised by the results.

Here are a few key verses about sleep:

**Psalm 3:5** - I lay down and slept; I awoke, for the Lord sustained me.

**Psalm 4:8** - I will both lie down in peace, and sleep; For You alone, O Lord, make me dwell in safety.

**Psalm 127:2** - It is in vain that you rise up early, to sit up late, to eat the bread of sorrows; for so He gives His beloved sleep.

**Proverbs 3:24** - When you lie down, you will not be afraid; Yes, you will lie down and your sleep will be sweet.

A few verses about stressing out and worrying:

**Matthew 11:28-30** - Come to Me, all who labour and are heavy laden, and I will give you rest. Take My yoke upon you, and learn from Me; for I am gentle and lowly in heart, and you will find rest for your souls. For My yoke is easy, and My burden is light.

**1 Peter 5:7** - Casting all your care upon Him, for He cares for you.

**John 14:27** - *Peace I leave with you,* My peace I give to you; not as the world gives do I give to you. Let not your heart be troubled, neither let it be afraid.

You don't need to have any faith or be religious to appreciate the theme of being at peace and unburdened. The gift of sleep is a precious blessing itself and a wonderful reminder that God is at work and that He loves and cares for us.

*As this is a book on sleep and not on faith then here are some universal affirmations and declarations on the following pages:*

## SLEEP AFFIRMATIONS

These are a great weapon on your armoury against insomnia. It could be argued that they are the most powerful, as our speech comes out as a vibrational frequency, and we all have our own unique voice-print. Some ancient manuscripts state that there is 'life and death in the power of the tongue'. Just look at children, and see how negative, intimidating and crushing words can ruin their lives; it's not called verbal abuse for nothing, as *it is abuse.* Contrast that with children who are praised for their works, achievements, and most importantly, for who they are as an individual person. They thrive, because someone *tells them* that they believe in them.

In an interesting Daily Mirror article, Dr Daisy Mae suggests that when settled in bed, keep your eyes open and try to deliberately stay awake as this will trick your mind into falling asleep. A phenomenon known as '*paradoxical intention*'. She also suggests repeating phrases such as, 'you must not fall asleep' or 'I will not fall asleep' so hopefully your eyes will tire and you'll fall asleep quickly (39).

Personally, I would never lie in bed at night and say 'I will not fall asleep' to myself. Ever. Do try the eyes wide open, staring at nothing trick if you like, as it could be a useful tool, but seriously consider whether it's wise to declare such negative statements over yourself. The last thing that you want to do is become a negative self-fulfilling prophecy.

However, there is a danger here that the power of the spoken word has not been considered. Most self-made millionaires know the power of the speaking out positive affirmations, and many will attribute such proactive affirmations to their success. It is not just the feeling of self-confidence but an overall feeling of wellbeing that can really eradicate any self-doubt.

If you are a naturally negative or pessimistic person, or if you thrive on self-depreciating humour then positive affirmations may seem a bit weird, but do give them a go, as they really can change your life. By positively reinforcing what we want to believe about ourselves we counteract the negative thoughts and feelings that we may have, therefore reducing stress and anxiety by default, which are often the main causes of insomnia anyway. They also allow you to be in the present moment, and letting go of negative thoughts can help your mind to relax.

**From the Bible to Buddha to Bruce Lee**

- Proverbs 23:7 For as he thinks in his heart, so is he.
- Buddha: The mind is everything. What you think, you become.
- Bruce Lee: As You Think, So Shall You Become.

Sleep affirmations can simply be read from a script, but aforementioned, there is power in the spoken word, and I would advise everyone to actually speak them out. They can be written on a postcard and kept as a bookmark, or displayed in a Perspex stand on your bedside table or on the wall next to your mirror as you brush your teeth. You could use the notepad on your phone or take a photo of a printed version, and you could always set a reminder on your phone or calendar to read them.

**Gratitude**

I am grateful for the safety of this room, the comfortable bed that I'll soon be asleep in, and the rest that it brings.

I am grateful to be able to rest, and for the gift of sleep, its restoration, and I welcome it now into my life.

**Self-worth**

I value and appreciate myself and I am worthy of a good night's sleep. Therefore, I let my mind completely relax because I deserve this natural gift.

**Release**

I choose to release all my worries, stress and tension and I let my body unwind, knowing that this will lead to a peaceful night's sleep.

I release any negative thoughts or feelings that may have occurred during the day, and I invite positive energy to rest inside of me.

**Peace & Love**

I am now at peace with myself and the world, so there is love and positivity around me and I drift off into a deep and nourishing sleep.

I choose to focus only on peaceful thoughts, as I am in control of my thoughts and my mind.

I am surrounded by love and positivity, even if it's not in those closest to me. Each day I attract more love, positivity and peace towards me.

I am able to manage whatever challenges life throws at me because I am becoming stronger each day and am able to handle the stresses and pressures of life.

I let go of any hurts or regrets of the past, and for today. I do not concern myself with tomorrow, for I cannot do anything about it now.

I drift off now, knowing that my heart is stilled, and that I am settled, and I have now put the cares of the world behind me. I believe that this sleep will repair my body and mind, and that I will wake up refreshed and ready for a brand-new day.

Feel free to cherry-pick a few, use them all, or use them as a guideline to create your own that are relevant to you. This is where knowing yourself and journaling is helpful, because you can target a particular worry or weakness and drive a positive affirmational sword right through it. They may sound a bit flowery or poncy but you will be amazed at what you can achieve by declaring affirmations out loud.

If you live alone, no problem, just get on with it. If you don't then consider working with your partner and reciting stuff together. If you do nothing more than laugh about it together then it's developed your relationship a little. If your partner is just, well, one of those, then you could recite the affirmations whilst in the bathroom at a push. Remember that you don't have to recite them perfectly each night; even just a basic acknowledgement in the bathroom is better than nothing.

This is your world, so you can choose whether to simply read or to recite. You can go through once or repeat several times. You could always visualise yourself in a peaceful and relaxing environment. Some say dozing in a canoe on a still lake. I like to think of being in a tent, as there could not be anyone or anything creeping up on me (as there could be on a beach), once inside it is relatively safe and all I can see is tent, so no distractions.

Try to be consistent and make it a part of your daily routine; you'll be more likely to see positive results. It may also take some time to for it to begin to feel normal, so be patient and give it a chance. If you've had a lifetime of negative thinking then that's unlikely to be cured in one evening, but keep at it and the results will come in time.

## EVENING ROUTINE

Our minds are not like light switches, they take a little time to unwind before switching off. Social media is rarely helpful in this final process. However, getting ready for bed may seem bland and formulaic, but if we're honest, much of our life actually is, and there's no harm in that. Hence why when returning from a fab holiday or having stayed over with friends/relatives you look forward to returning to the comfort and humdrum of your normal home life. Think of your average morning routine between waking up and leaving your home on a normal working day. You went through all the motions to get ready as part of your routine; it is what it is, so having a night-time routine is not as weird or ritualistic as people may think.

We are often in a heightened level of alertness, and tech seems to keep us there, with rings, buzzes and pings permeating our lives to the extent of never really winding down properly, as we're on permanent standby for the latest notification, which is a bit of a passion killer. Everyone's bedtime and wind-down time is different. The more you struggle to either get to sleep or stay asleep the more important a good wind-down session becomes, so just be aware of consuming too much media before you go to bed.

The new buzzword or sleep method is called cognitive shuffle, which is when you're settled and ready to sleep you start to think of a random word, say, 'sleeping' and then think of as many words that begin with 's' and really picture each one, e.g., snowman, sandcastle, snot, etc., then move onto the next original word letter of 'l' and so on. This apparently keeps your brain occupied enough that you're not worrying about the mortgage, your diet, money etc. and it tires your brain out enough to fall asleep. Keep the pictures meaningless though, otherwise it could snap you back into alertness. Just be aware that when your partner whispers you the question of *'what you thinking about right now?'* that 'an aardvark' is a pretty bizarre response. Better to say 'you dear' and leave it at that. I see the benefits of the cognitive shuffle, but my magnificent mind is way too random. I'd rather brainstorm my thoughts onto paper or do a crossword to tire myself out. Try both, and see what happens.

Electronic devices are often seen as the villains of successful slumber, but it is possible to make them work for you rather than against you. You can turn your phone to flight mode and still use sleep apps, white noise and alarms, yet you won't be distracted by texts or notifications. The brightness of an iPad or Kindle can be reduced, and font size can be increased, therefore making text easier to read, and potentially using less ambient lighting than what is required for reading a book. Podcasts and meditations can both assist with relaxation, so tech can be useful.

An important point to note is that *worrying* about using your phone before sleep can be worse than actually *going* on your phone. If you start thinking that you won't sleep because you've just been on your phone right before bed then you probably won't sleep so well. Trust me, worrying about anything is usually worse than the actual thing itself.

Preparing for beddy-byes can be made into a calming ritual without getting overly weird about it. Try a few simple things like:

- Dimming the household lights which will help your mind wind down. No dimmer switches? No problem; use smaller table lights. Salt lamps supposedly reduce 'digital haze', clean the air and reduce asthma and allergies. Practically they do give a lovely soft glow to a room and are perfect for children's bedrooms that need a nightlight.
- Try lighting a nice candle, ideally unscented (like a church candle or beeswax) or buy an expensive scented one. If you go for the pound-shop nasties then they are sure to have

been made with dubious chemicals. Candles can be part of your settling down process. Their soft glow makes naked bodies look far nicer too.

- Throw out any plug-in air fresheners from your house. They give me headaches and in my opinion, they are lethal. They cause ENT problems; they are a man-made chemical that has been aromatised and is being breathed in. They are endocrine disrupters, cause neurotoxicity and may cause cancers (40). So get rid!
- Listening to calming music, relaxation podcasts or audio books. Whale 'music' must get a mention here, as it appears to be the epitome of relaxation therapy.
- A ticking clock may settle you down and provide reassurance to help you nod off. However, you could be reminded, second by second, that there are 3600 of them per hour, so they're not for everyone. If not for you then the good news is that you can buy non-ticking clocks or non-ticking mechanisms for your regular clock to avoid this.
- Use a nice room spray within 30 minutes before bed and after a day or so the smell will trigger your 'settling down' phase. Smells can be very powerful for establishing habits and relaxing. Don't believe me? Pick a flower of whatever reminds you of your childhood and have a smell. The smell will take you right back to your childhood (only in memory, flowers are not time machines).
- Lavender is hardly the panacea of all sleeping woes, yet everyone seems to recommend this herby fragrance. I am totally happy with associating the smell of lavender with being relaxed and feeling sleepy. Associating lavender with sleep forms a mental trigger for me to relax whenever I smell it. If you're not there yet then fake it until you make it. Marks & Spencer do a nice 3-in-1 room/linen/body spray which is

light and delicate enough. If you're a fan of Laura Ashley and Cottagecore then lavender is definitely for you.

- Television has now found its way into people's bedrooms, but I must remind myself that this is the $21^{st}$ century. Personally, I think that bedrooms should only be for reading, sleeping or expressing sexuality. However, the TV does have some redeeming features such as nature or travel documentaries which can be very relaxing, and I've even used them to send my children to sleep before carrying them up to bed. Sir David Attenborough has a very melodious and soothing vice. It is generally best to avoid Jerry Springer though.
- Try doing some form of meditation, breath-work, or general relaxation. Do a breath-sprint, where you breathe in and out as fast as you can for 10-60 seconds. Try it, it will certainly release some tensions. Start with 5-10 breaths and see how you feel.
- Unwind your body with a simple stretching routine. It really does reduce physical tension and will help to keep you supple. And young. And fresh. If you actually do it.
- Showering/bathing, massage (self-massage can be surprisingly powerful and healing, just massage the areas that you can reach, and accept the ones that you can't). You don't need fancy massage oil, olive or coconut oil will do.
- Reflecting/journalling. Journalling is one of those things that seem so lame to those who don't do it, yet those who do it seem to swear by it. If journalling is the one key thing that helps you sleep by unwinding your mind, evaluating your general progress in life and provide structure for your future then do it. It can be a very useful tool.
- Having a light bite to eat and a tisane (herbal tea) can help settle your tummy to avoid waking up hungry. Moderation and balance are key here.

- If you've spent evening after evening working on your sleep routine and you're still awake then throw all the routines out and do what you enjoy; at least you'll feel more fulfilled. Often a simple hobby can be enough to provide some enjoyment and the reward of achievement. Too many people think that a personal hobby is a bit lame or that they haven't got time, but by cutting back on all things media it is surprising how much more time becomes available. If the hobby becomes the one thing that de-stresses and sufficiently relaxes you for sleep then it really is beneficial. Consider going through your photographs that are on memory sticks somewhere, print them off and cut them up to make a collage that you can put into a photo frame. You can pick frames up for next to nothing if you get creative. There you go, your new hobby!

**The curved ball**: try doing a set of deep breathing exercises at some point during your day. Be creative, they can easily be hidden from work colleagues, and be incorporated somewhere into your daily schedule. The easiest way to avoid embarrassment at home or work is to have it out in the open, so depending on your work environment you could get your colleagues on board and have a quick 10 deep breaths challenge. Ditto some basic stretches throughout the day.

Private or public, you won't arrive home quite so knotted up and require so much 'me-time' in order to de-stress. Reducing daily stresses should be a general lifestyle approach, not something that is crammed into your evening routine.

# FINAL SUMMARY

- Buy the best quality bed, mattress, pillows, bedding that you can afford. Consider requesting such as gifts for birthdays and Christmas. Do try different fabrics and pillows; utilise hotels where possible and ask questions about bed types. Remember that you'd look great in a Scrooge nightgown and sleeping cap.
- Make sure your bedroom environment is sleep-friendly. Ensure that it is cool, dark, quiet and well-ventilated where possible. Keep it dust free and minimal; deal with your floordrobe! Utilise accessories such as eye masks, earplugs, white noise and/or light machines etc.
- Try to get as much exposure to natural light as possible. Reduce screentime in the evenings to avoid blue light. Aim to turn off your electronic devices at least an hour before bed to give your mind time to unwind. Keep your bedroom only for sleep and intimacy. Therefore, avoid using your bed for work, studying, or watching TV. This helps train your brain to associate the bedroom with sleep.
- Address any underlying sleep disorders. Monitoring your sleep with tech can provide data to help, but don't get caught up with analysis-paralysis. However, tech can be a good tool to discover anomalies. If you suspect you do have a sleep disorder, such as sleep apnoea or genuine long-term insomnia then consult a healthcare professional for a proper evaluation and treatment.
- Try natural sleep aids such as herbal teas, melatonin supplements, or lavender aromatherapy, and re-read the Chemical Cosh disclaimers for advice on what I can't condone.
- Establish a consistent sleep schedule. Try to go to bed and wake up at the same time every day, even on weekends. Allow for variables though; don't be too retentive about it.

- Create a relaxing bedtime routine. Engage in activities that promote relaxation, such as reading a book, taking a warm bath, or practising meditation. You may have to miss some 'great' TV or getting up to level 9 in World of Warcraft, so remember that you are doing this as a de-stressing treat for yourself.
- Try to avoid the legal drugs of caffeine, nicotine, and alcohol too close to bedtime as they can interfere with your sleep. Reduce your intake of fluids as the evening progresses, to minimise nocturnal lavatorial expeditions.
- If you need to take a nap then try to keep it short (around 5-60 minutes) and avoid napping too close to bedtime. Find what works for you, but don't become too reliant on them.
- Regular physical activity can help to promote better sleep. Ideally it's 30 minutes per day; realistically just try to do as much as you can on most days of the week. Avoid vigorous exercise too close to bedtime
- Avoid heavy meals before bedtime to avoid discomfort, indigestion and the night sweats; try to have your last meal a few hours before you go to sleep.
- Find healthy ways to manage your stress. This can be part of your wind-down process but it can also be blowing off steam in the evenings, or simply doing something that you enjoy, such as a hobby.
- Practise relaxation techniques, such as deep breathing, progressive muscle relaxation, or self-affirmations using guided imagery to relax your mind and body before sleep. If you don't fall asleep within 20-40 minutes then get out of bed and engage in a relaxing or meaningful activity until you feel sleepy again. Be aware that constantly checking the time can create anxiety and make it harder to fall asleep.

This entire book has been about finding what works the best for you, so it may take some trial and error to find the right sleep conquering strategies.

# CONCLUSION

Live like your great-grandparents. Life was hard, but social life was good (and meaningful; *people talked to each other*). Look at pictures of families in their homes and gardens from the 1920s-1970s. They didn't have a lot of stuff, and yet there was a sense of contentment from spending time with each other. The physical work was harder for both men and women and people probably slept a lot better for it. In the pre-tech eras people used to go for a stroll after their evening meal which helped settle the mind ready for bed, and provided meaningful social interaction. Their minds were not bombarded with advertisements from the media nor the internet.

Cosmetic surgery or celebrity obsession was not a part of that culture, and today we are drowning in a sea of information overload. The internet is such a crazy encyclopaedia of knowledge, which can be very helpful and useful, but like fire, it is a good servant but a bad master. I'm more cautious now of what internet rabbit holes that I go down in the evening. Our televisions are *programming* us to believe what the people controlling the news and the *programmes* want us to believe. Smartphones are a bit of a double-edged sword for the modern person. We all know the benefits but they can be a *huge* waste of time. In the 21st century we have more gadgets to save time and yet we still seem so busy and lacking in time. I coined the phrase last year: *'The more entertainment we have, the less entertained we are'.*

Of all things, a humble book can help to slow our minds down (or at least, not overload them) and they tire our eyes out without information overload. This can block off some of life's pressures and help to settle us ready for bed. For those who say that they don't really read should evaluate what they are doing on their phones. Unless they are watching endless TikTok or playing Candy Crush then they are probably reading something, so swap the screen for a book and save your eyes and rest your mind. Magazines bridge the gap for the hardcore phone addicts, or perhaps consider reading the Beano. If this book has bored you to sleep then please do not give it a negative review, for it has achieved its purpose by default.

There should be enough information in this book to provide you with sufficient solutions to tackle the pain of insomnia. However, now that you are here, do try to implement what you have read, and be cautious about moving on to the next sleep article or book like a flitting bird. Being obsessed about insomnia rarely leads to better sleep, and quite often, the opposite is true. So, implement what you've learnt here and go and read something more interesting when you're sleeping better. One cream cake won't make you morbidly obese, and missing one evening of your relaxation ritual won't necessarily give you a bad night. Unless you lie awake worrying that it might.

There is a danger that with all our routines and excessive sleep hygiene, with issues such as lights, blackouts, tech and WIFI off, supper, candles, ra-de-ra can make us unable to sleep anywhere else. That said, many of us sleep better when away due to leaving all our troubles behind. Also, don't feel pressured to download all the apps or get every sleep analysis gadget going. For people who are prone to worry, not knowing the data may be better. Some of the modern technology is very beneficial, but if you are wallowing in the quagmire of analysis paralysis then it may not work for you. These are great tools to give you a baseline of how you sleep, so that you can track your improvements and get help if necessary. Although I've not tried all of the technology and gadgets, I've done sufficient research whilst writing this to state that everything in here has had good reviews. Items within this book may not be the most exciting present to give or to receive, but if chosen carefully and used daily, they will be a very thoughtful and practical gift.

I have tried all the sleeping methods at some point, but I remain flexible with my nightly routine, and yes, sometimes I'm still doom-scrolling just before lights out. It is what it is, we all have a life. However, a general sort of wind-down is worth it, especially not clogging up my mind with information overload. I've stopped trying to cram everything in before bedtime, but to work harder on days off during the day to enable more relaxing and settled evenings.

We cannot force our sleep and it cannot be controlled. There really isn't a one size fits all solution for our lifestyles. Even the most steadfast routine has its variables. At best, we can take positive steps to avoid stresses, relax our bodies and minds by winding down. Sleep is a passive process, like digestion. Sometimes by stopping our obsession of getting more sleep it will naturally follow; but like all the best plans, not always, so keep trying and be blessed.

# REFERENCES


1) https://www.cdc.gov/sleep/about_sleep/chronic_disease.html
2) https://jcsm.aasm.org/doi/full/10.5664/jcsm.6472
3) https://www.matalan.co.uk/homeware/bedroom/bedroom-buyers-guide/duvet-filling-and-tog-guide
4) https://www.researchgate.net/publication/243970419_A_Systematic_Review_Assessing_Bidirectionality_between_Sleep_Disturbances_Anxiety_and_Depression
5) https://rowlandearthing.co.uk/pages/science
6) https://www.health.harvard.edu/staying-healthy/blue-light-has-a-dark-side
7) https://www.mattressadvisor.com/should-you-be-sleeping-naked/
8) https://www.sciencedaily.com/releases/2022/06/220606181217.htm
9) https://www.dovepress.com/sleep-positions-and-nocturnal-body-movements-based-on-free-living-acce-peer-reviewed-fulltext-article-NSS
10) https://www.mayoclinic.org/diseases-conditions/snoring/diagnosis-treatment/drc-20377701
11) https://medlineplus.gov/ency/presentations/100038_4.htm
12) https://tucked.co.uk/stages-of-sleep/
13) https://www.cdc.gov/media/releases/2016/p0215-enough-sleep.html
14) https://www.medscape.org/viewarticle/585753
15) https://www.cdc.gov/sleep/about_sleep/how_much_sleep.html

16) https://www.guinnessworldrecords.com/news/2023/1/whats-the-limit-to-how-long-a-human-can-stay-awake-733188
17) https://en.wikipedia.org/wiki/Continuous_positive_airway_pressure
18) Polysomnogram Image By 邱鈺鋒 - Own work, CC BY-SA 4.0, https://commons.wikimedia.org/w/index.php?curid=58305846
19) https://en.wikipedia.org/wiki/Sleepwalking
20) https://www.manchestereveningnews.co.uk/news/greater-manchester-news/road-ban-for-prestwich-gp-who-863592
21) https://www.nhs.uk/conditions/sleepwalking/
22) https://www.nhs.uk/conditions/sleep-paralysis/
23) https://en.wikipedia.org/wiki/Sleep_paralysis
24) https://www.nhs.uk/conditions/narcolepsy/
25) https://en.wikipedia.org/wiki/%CE%93-Aminobutyric_acid
26) https://www.ncbi.nlm.nih.gov/books/NBK526132/
27) https://en.wikipedia.org/wiki/Amygdala
28) https://www.drinkaware.co.uk/facts/health-effects-of-alcohol/effects-on-the-body/alcohol-and-sleep
29) Helmanis L (2019) Clean Sleeping: How to Sleep Better Naturally Carlton, London
30) https://www.rospa.com/road-safety/advice/roads/clock-change
31) Law.G (2017) Sleep Better Sheldon Press. London
32) https://www.google.com/search?client=firefox-b-d&q=when+were+bells+attatched+to+people+buried+in+a+graveyard%3F
33) Leschziner G (2019) The Secret World of Sleep Simon & Schuster London
34) https://www.bmj.com/content/363/bmj.k4641
35) https://myvision.org/eye-conditions/eyelash-mites/

36) https://www.healthline.com/nutrition/banana-before-bed
37) https://health.clevelandclinic.org/i-sigh-a-lot-what-does-that-mean/
38) https://www.google.com/search?client=firefox-b-d&q=does+a+yawn+or+sigh+relaease+dopamine
39) https://www.mirror.co.uk/news/weird-news/doctor-shares-unusual-open-eye-29004958
40) https://www.google.com/search?q=dangers+of+plug+in+air+fresheners&client=firefox9p
41) https://www.youtube.com/watch?v=nrRklKnehIs Sleeping on the Floor
42) https://www.youtube.com/watch?v=YP1M8JjKx2Y Sleeping on the Floor

## SLEEP GOALS

| Page No. | What I want to achieve | Time-scale: 1-8 weeks | Results/ Evaluation |
|---|---|---|---|
| | | | |
| | | | |
| | | | |
| | | | |
| | | | |
| | | | |
| | | | |
| | | | |

# THE EPWORTH SLEEPINESS SCALE

- No chance of dozing =0
- Slight chance of dozing =1
- Moderate chance of dozing =2
- High chance of dozing =3

Write down the number corresponding to your choice in the right-hand column. Total your score below.

| SITUATION | CHANCE OF DOZING |
|---|---|
| Sitting and reading | |
| Watching TV | |
| Sitting inactive in a public place (e.g., a theatre or a meeting) | |
| As a passenger in a car for an hour without a break | |
| Lying down to rest in the afternoon when circumstances permit | |
| Sitting and talking to someone | |
| Sitting quietly after a lunch without alcohol | |
| In a car, while stopped for a few minutes in traffic | |

Total Score = ____________________________

**Analyse Your Score**

**Interpretation:**

**0-7**: It is unlikely that you are abnormally sleepy.
**8-9:** You have an average amount of daytime sleepiness.
**10-15**: You may be excessively sleepy depending on the situation. You may want to consider
seeking medical attention.
**16-24**: You are excessively sleepy and should consider seeking medical attention.

*Reference: Johns MW. A new method for measuring daytime sleepiness: The Epworth Sleepiness Scale. Sleep 1991; 14(6):540-5.*

# SLEEP CHART

| | Mon | Tue | Wed | Thur | Fri | Sat | Sun |
|---|---|---|---|---|---|---|---|
| Energy or mood during the day | | | | | | | |
| Last activity before bed | | | | | | | |
| Medications<br>Supplements | | | | | | | |
| Last time and type of food | | | | | | | |
| Last time and type of drink | | | | | | | |
| Alcohol | | | | | | | |
| Bedtime | | | | | | | |

| | | | | | | | |
|---|---|---|---|---|---|---|---|
| Lights out | | | | | | | |
| Hours asleep | | | | | | | |
| How many times awake | | | | | | | |
| Toilet breaks | | | | | | | |
| Time awake in morning | | | | | | | |
| Awoke refreshed? | | | | | | | |
| | | | | | | | |

For medication/supplements just list any changes; you don't need to write down your regulars every day, and use initials or symbols to save writing. The blank boxes could be used for expressing sexuality, or variables, such as if snoring woke you up etc. You could also make your own table using these ideas, or add your own that are relevant to you. Don't overthink it, rough data is all that you need. Remember to always date the charts, you'll be glad that you did when reflecting back.

Printed in Great Britain
by Amazon

26231003R00116